365

ways to turn him on

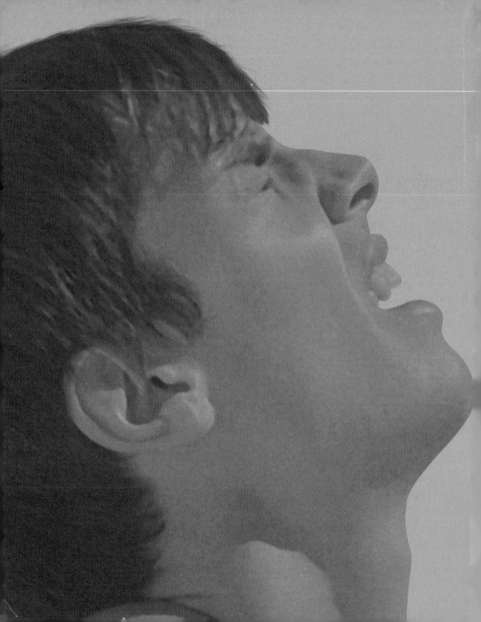

365

ways to turn him on

DK would like to thank lovehoney.co.uk for providing lingerie, toys, costumes, and other fun things. The items featured in the book, along with many others, are available to order from their website.

LOVEH♥NEY.co.uk

Many thanks to John Rowley (photographer), Russell Burton (assistant to photographer), Kat Mead (photography direction), Peter Mallory (photography production), and Enzo Volpe (hair and make-up). Thank you to Clare Hubbard for proofreading and Laura Mingozzi for design assistance.

Special thanks to Kesta Desmond.

Contents

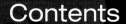

Q: What's the best way to turn on a man?

A: Give him more than a hard-on. Do something that makes his whole body tingle… something that gets his mind burning as hotly as his rod… something that turns him from a grown man into a lust-addled teenager.

How do you do this?

It's simple—take a tour of the following 183 pages. Pick from a dizzying array of irresistibly sexy turn-on techniques. You'll find everything from the sensually sweet at one end to the seriously wicked at the other.

So grab his hand and pull him into the bedroom. Whether you turn him to putty with your fingertips or shock him with a kinky roleplay, don't stop until he's on his knees and cross-eyed with desire.

And… if, after days of taking him to the high peaks of desire, you fancy a trip up there yourself, it's easy. Just close this book, turn it upside-down and pop it under your lover's pillow. He'll soon get the picture.

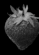

When the mood is sweet and sensual

Turn-ons to make him melt all over

When the mood is hot and erotic

Turn-ons to make him crazy with lust

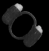

When the mood is rude and raunchy

Turn-ons to bring out his naughty side

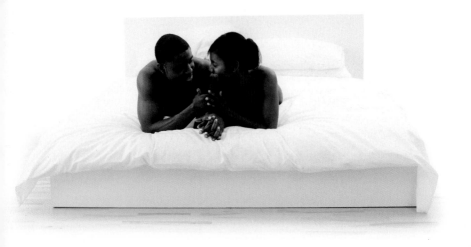

Twine your hand in his, look into his eyes, and pay him a loving compliment.

Perfect for: Giving him hot flutters in his heart and crotch.
Irresistible when: Your hands slip down his body with depravity in mind.

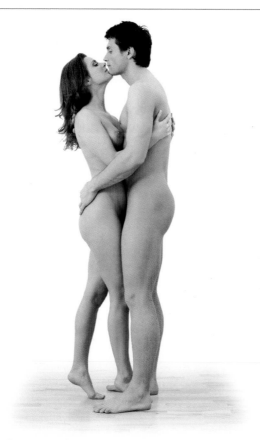

Rest your chin against his, so you're almost kissing.

Perfect for: Giving him an erotic will-we-or-won't-we frisson.
Irresistible when: You take the lead, and decide you will.

363 Tugging his arm

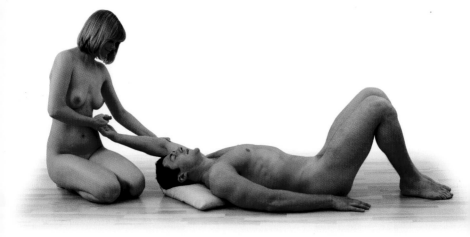

Hold his hand in yours, grip him above the elbow, and gently pull his arm.

Perfect for: A sensual stretch that ripples all the way down his spine.
Irresistible when: You glide your hands, palm over palm, along his arm.

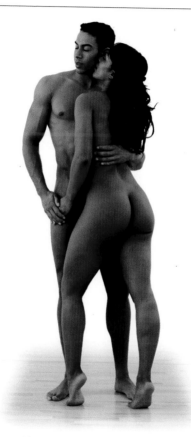

Kiss him tenderly along his jawline.

Perfect for: A blissful glow that spreads across his whole face.
Irresistible when: You take the tip of his ear lobe in your mouth, and suck gently.

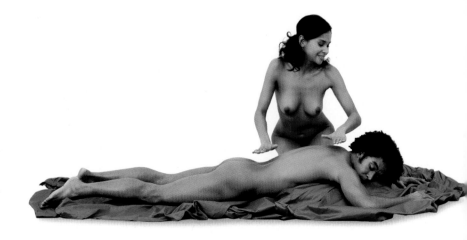

Hold your hands a short distance from his body, and massage his energy field.

Perfect for: Making him feel radiant and glowing.
Irresistible when: You roll him over, and charge his love wand.

Love blanket 360

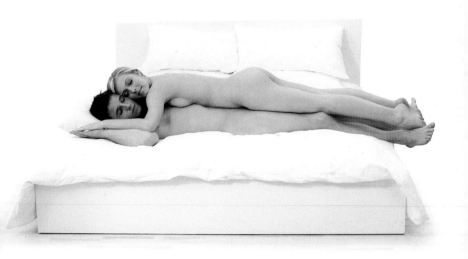

Perfectly mold your body to his.

Perfect for: Intense, bonding moments.
Irresistible when: You gyrate your hips in slow motion.

359 Bumpy-rumpy

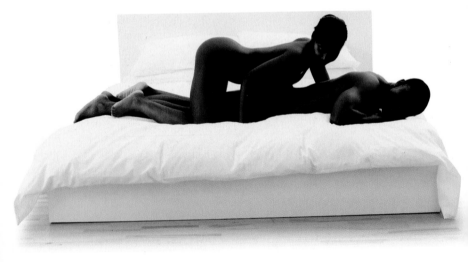

Glide your oiled bumps over his smooth rump.

Perfect for: When he's in need of a heavenly caress.
Irresistible when: You carry on up to enclose his face in your rising beauties.

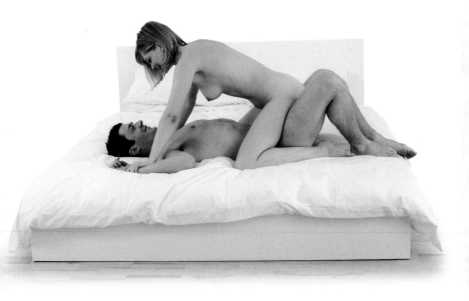

Straddle him, and pin his wrists to the bed.

Perfect for: When he's in the mood to be taken.
Irresistible when: You tease him until he's ready to blow.

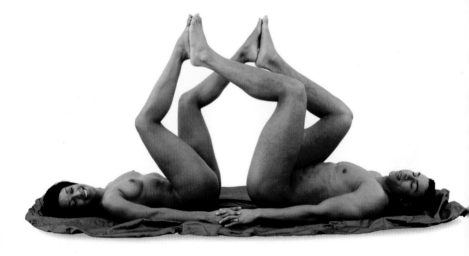

Lie on your back, and press your feet against his—now pedal.

Perfect for: Titillating friction on his helmet.
Irresistible when: You get tired, and have to grab his handlebar.

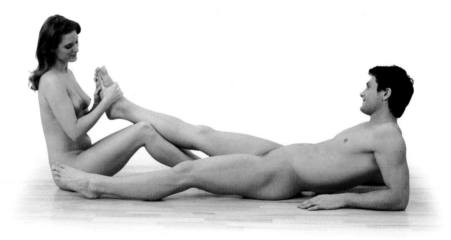

Take his foot in your hands, and press your thumbs in firm circles on the sole.

Perfect for: Making him moan out loud with pleasure.
Irresistible when: You massage, kiss, and caress your way up his whole body.

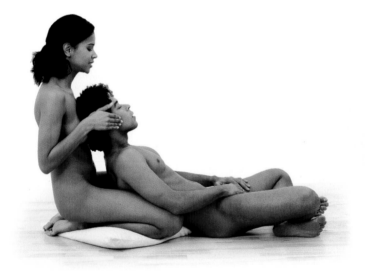

Circle your fingertips on his temples, and along his jaw line.

Perfect for: Unplugging his brain, and enveloping him in waves of bliss.
Irresistible when: You softly stroke his whole face.

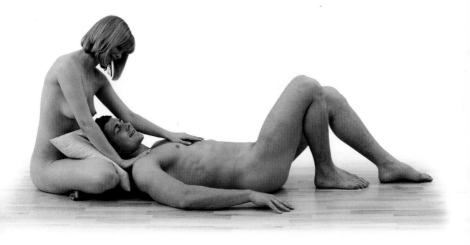

Use your hands to press, rub, knead, and rake his shoulders and chest.

Perfect for: Letting him surrender to pure sensuality.
Irresistible when: You tell him what a gorgeous body he has.

353 Trouser teaser

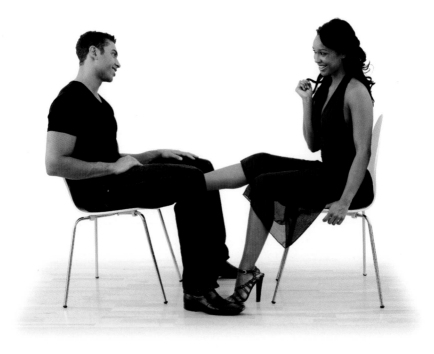

While chatting, slip off your shoe, and "rest" your foot between his legs.

Perfect for: Making him writhe with horniness.
Irresistible when: You take the conversation in a filthy direction.

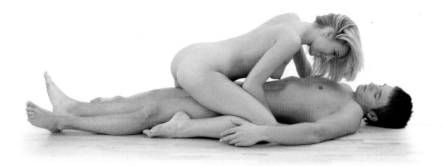

Straddle his body, and tickle his skin with your locks.

Perfect for: Making him shiver with lust.
Irresistible when: You lean in, and brush your nipples against him.

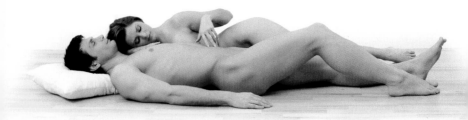

Softly trail your fingertips over his belly and chest.

Perfect for: When you want to tease, and arouse him sensually.
Irresistible when: Your fingertip tour extends to his joystick.

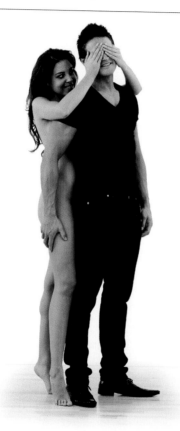

Sneak up, and cover his eyes when he comes through the door.

Perfect for: Sending lightning-fast tingles of anticipation from brain to crotch.
Irresistible when: You get him into bed, and delight him with sheer sluttishness.

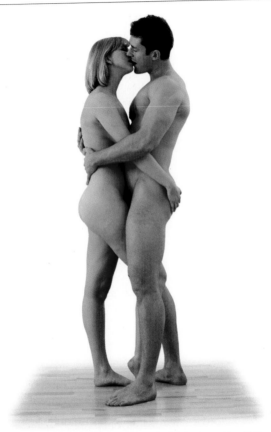

Grab his buttocks, and pull him in tight as you kiss him.

Perfect for: The voluptuous pressure of your belly against his pole.
Irresistible when: You slip your hand between your bodies.

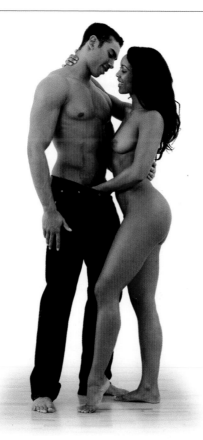

Take advantage mid-smooch, and slip your hand discreetly into his jeans.

Perfect for: When there's a risk of being caught.
Irresistible when: You provide some cover by pressing your body close to his.

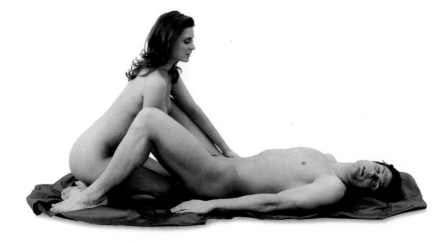

Massage the sensitive super-spot halfway between his balls and anus.

Perfect for: Intensely pleasurable strokes that ripple to his prostate.
Irresistible when: You stroke his perineum, and his erection at the same time.

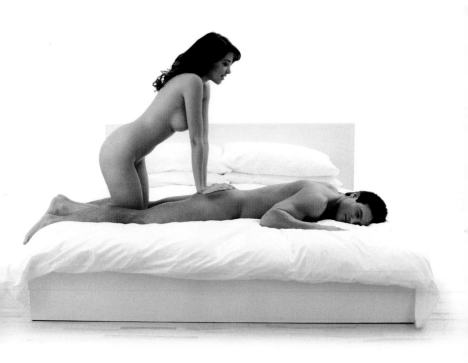

Lean deeply into his buttock muscles—as though pushing him through the bed.

Perfect for: A glow that starts in his butt, and radiates throughout the region.
Irresistible when: You give him hot, pelvic vibrations by jiggling your hands.

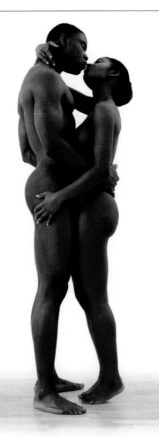

Stand with your lips a hair's breadth away from his mouth.

Perfect for: Filling him with a fierce yearning to taste you.
Irresistible when: You caress his lips with cool, minty breath.

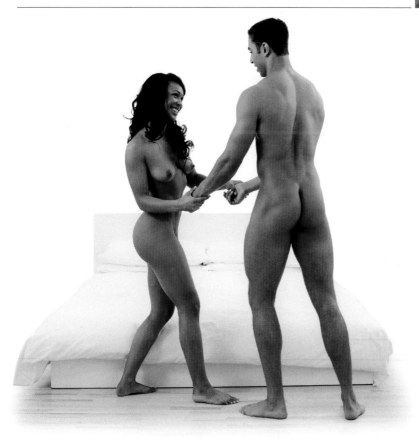

Grab his wrists, and pull him onto the bed.

Perfect for: Times when he thinks he's too busy.
Irresistible when: You brush your soft, smooth, kissable body against him.

343 Palm-to-palm

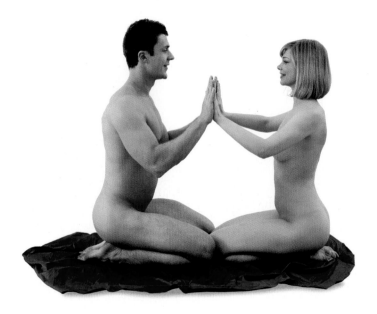

Give him loving energy by pressing your palms against his. Gaze into his eyes.

Perfect for: Amazing him with the slow-burning bliss of Tantra.
Irresistible when: You anoint his sacred parts with massage oil.

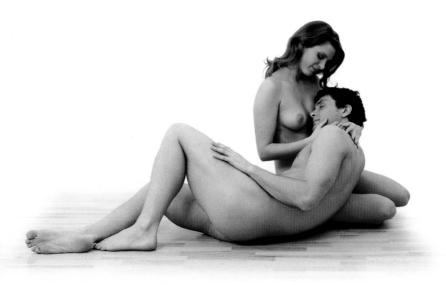

Cradle his head in your arms as he lies in your lap.

Perfect for: Taking away all his cares with sweet, loving tenderness.
Irresistible when: You shower him with soft kisses.

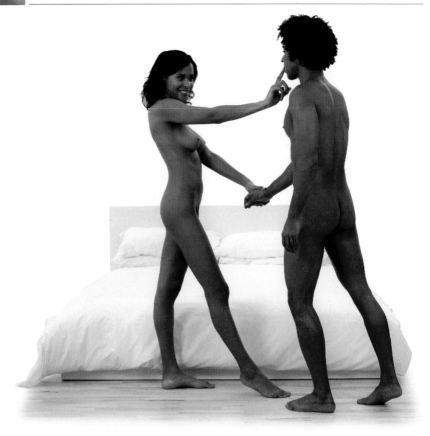

Tease him with a restraining finger when he's ready to pounce.

Perfect for: Creating incendiary lust.
Irresistible when: You give yourself to him one erotic step at a time.

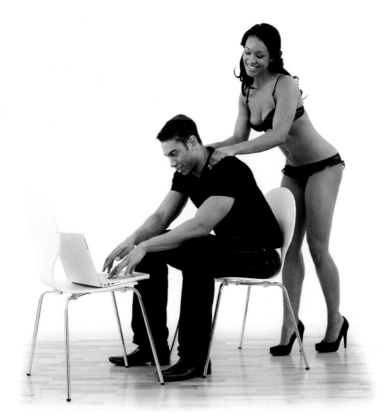

Lure him away from work with a penetrating shoulder rub—and some killer lingerie.

Perfect for: Pressing fingers and thumbs deeply into his "Ahhhhhh" spots.
Irresistible when: You smooth your hands over his back, and kiss his neck.

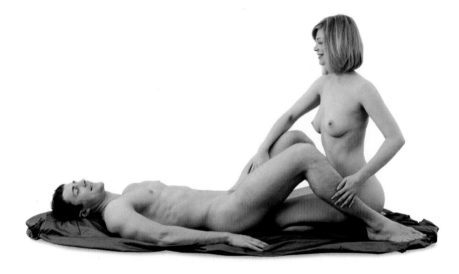

Trace a meandering line with your fingertips along his inner thigh.

Perfect for: Making his knees tremble with anticipation.
Irresistible when: Your fingers pause to admire the size of his peak.

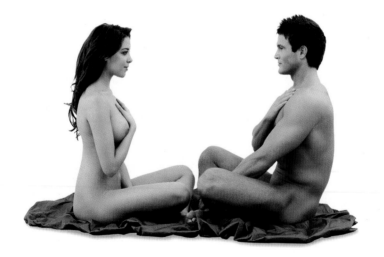

Ask him to put his hand on his heart, and gaze into your soul.

Perfect for: Getting high on loving union.
Irresistible when: You kiss him with reverent sensuality.

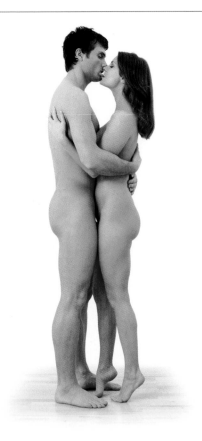

Take his lower lip between yours. Gently suck and nibble.

Perfect for: Making his skin prickle with anticipation.
Irresistible when: You follow it up with your warm, soft tongue on his love stack.

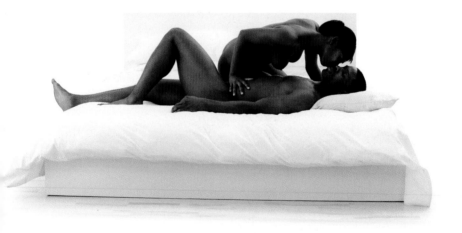

Sprinkle his face with loving kisses before he opens his eyes.

Perfect for: The sensual beginning to a day in bed.
Irresistible when: You let your hands drift softly over his skin.

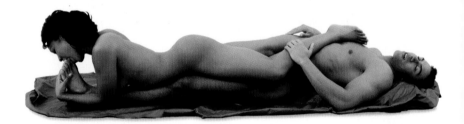

Drink something hot, then slip your lips over his toes and suck.

Perfect for: Scorching sensations to make him melt.
Irresistible when: You wiggle your hips to start a fire in his groin.

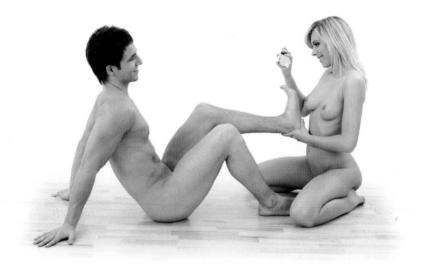

Take his foot in your hand, and drizzle edible oil onto his toes.

Perfect for: De-stressing him at the end of the day.
Irresistible when: You sprinkle each toe with licks and kisses.

333 Getting him well oiled

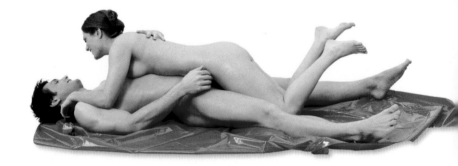

Lie on a PVC sheet, and get him slick with oil, then swim on his body.

Perfect for: Helpless pleasure as he submits to your slippery softness.
Irresistible when: You writhe against each other with abandon.

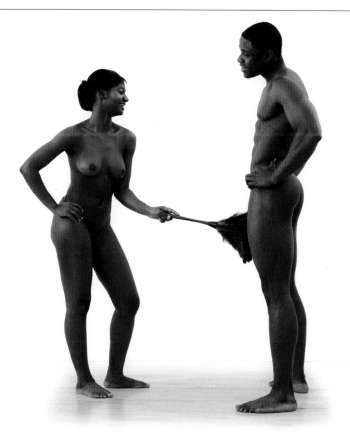

Take a fluffy feather duster, and waft it over his treasures.

Perfect for: Putting a grin on his face, and a shine on his scepter.
Irresistible when: You offer him a special spit-and-polish service too.

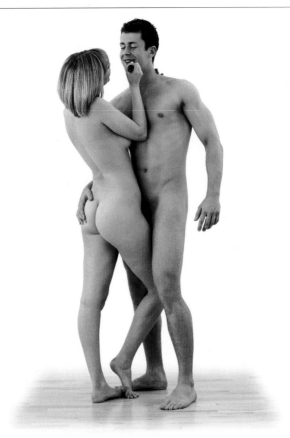

Bring out his feminine side—paint him with your lipstick.

Perfect for: Going to a cross-dressing party.
Irresistible when: You kiss it all off him.

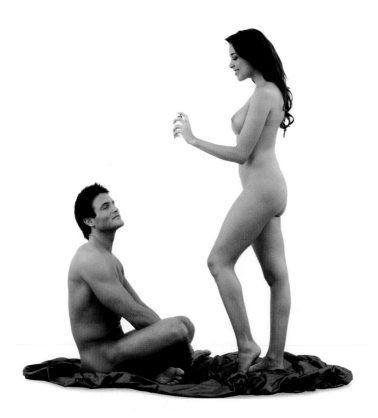

Let a delicate spray of your perfume land on his face.

Perfect for: A sensual opening to a night of romance.
Irresistible when: You move closer, and let him taste as well as smell you.

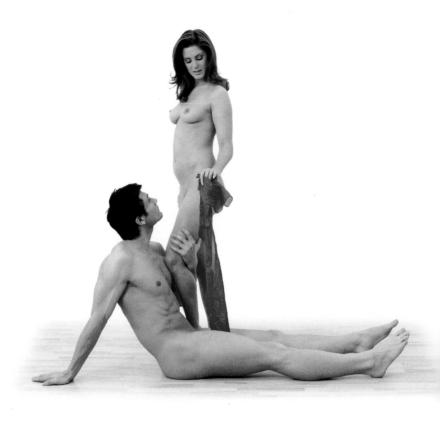

Waft a silk scarf across his flagpole.

Perfect for: Letting him bask in subtle sensuality.
Irresistible when: You blindfold him with the scarf, then do something wicked.

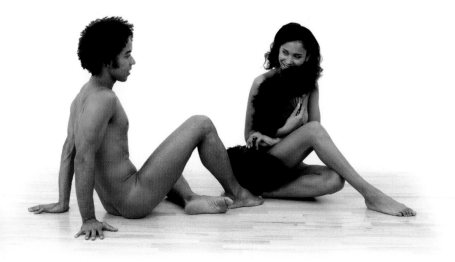

Hide your best assets behind a fan or two.

Perfect for: Lighting his fuse, flamenco-style.
Irresistible when: You offer to play his castanets afterward.

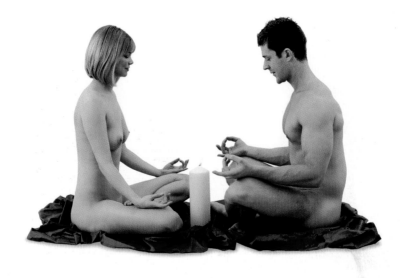

Have your wick-ed way with him—meditate on a candle flame before you touch.

Perfect for: Leaving the world behind, and making him feel at one with you.
Irresistible when: You stroke his face, and gaze lovingly into his eyes.

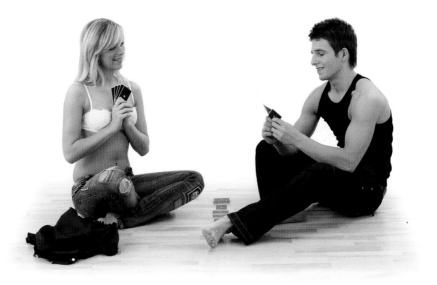

Challenge him to a game of strip poker.

Perfect for: A second-date seduction.
Irresistible when: You just keep getting a losing hand…

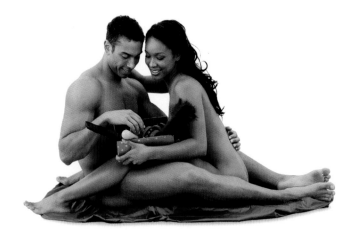

Ask him to take his pick from a box of erotic props and tools.

Perfect for: Firing him up with erotic inspiration.
Irresistible when: You take the toy of his choice, and give him an X-rated demo.

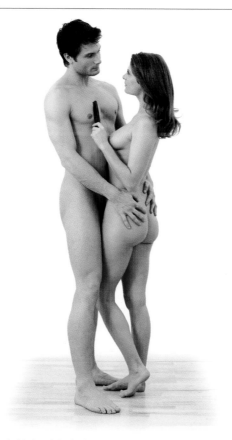

Gently comb his body hair. If he hasn't got any, rake his skin instead.

Perfect for: Giving him that intimately groomed feeling.
Irresistible when: You teasingly ruffle his pubes.

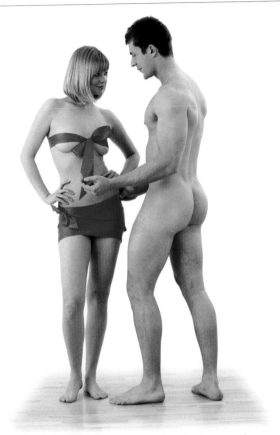

Wrap yourself in ribbons, and tell him "I'm yours".

Perfect for: Triggering his want-you-naked-now urge.
Irresistible when: You put the end of the ribbon between his teeth.

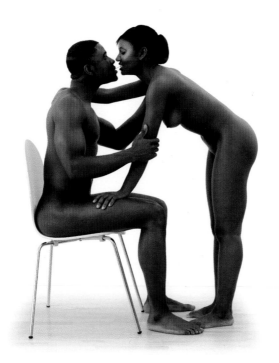

Lean over, and share your strip of chewing gum with him.

Perfect for: Flirtiness that brings you breathtakingly close.
Irresistible when: You close the gap, and slip each other the tongue.

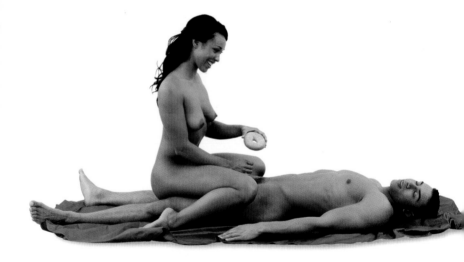

Make him feel delectable—push a warm doughnut over his manhood.

Perfect for: When he knows you never say "No" to sweets.
Irresistible when: You lick the sugar from his ring with torturous slowness.

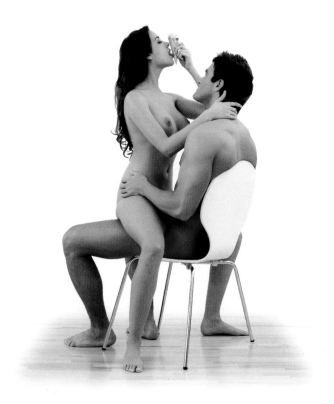

Pretend you're in an ice-cream ad—lick the drips with orgasmic enthusiasm.

Perfect for: Making him crave your tongue on his cone.
Irresistible when: You devour every trace of ice cream, then head south.

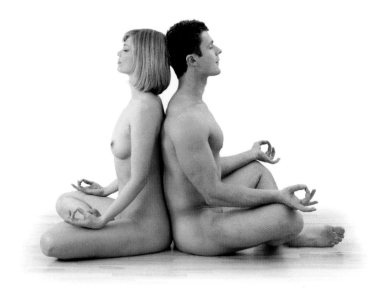

Sit back to back, and ask him to raise his kundalini.

Perfect for: Making his chakras spin with sexy anticipation.
Irresistible when: You give him a tingling, Tantric massage afterward.

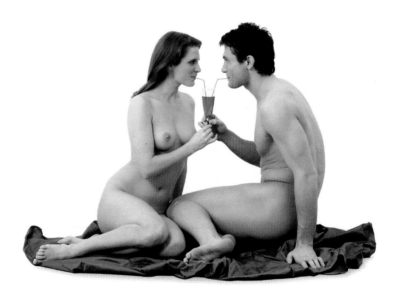

Pop a straw in his cocktail, and help him suck.

Perfect for: Sending a cheeky "I want you" message at parties.
Irresistible when: You kiss him lingeringly on the cheek when the glass is empty.

317 Sucking up to him

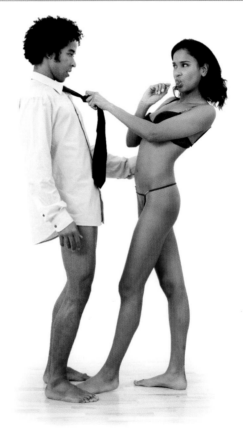

Use a lollipop to show off your tongue-twirling skills.

Perfect for: Giving him red-hot fantasies about where he wants your lips.
Irresistible when: You slowly unwrap his candy stick.

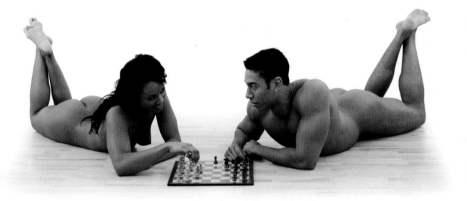

Thrash him in a naked game of chess.

Perfect for: When he likes having his castle crushed and his bishop bashed.
Irresistible when: You give new meaning to "I'm putting you in checkmate".

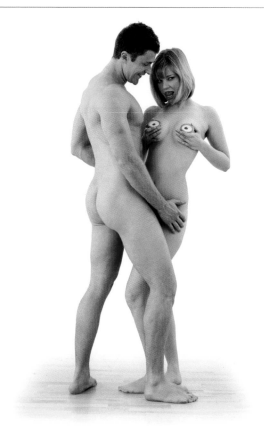

Sidle up, and ask him if he likes your cupcakes.

Perfect for: When he wants to have his cake, and eat it.
Irresistible when: You finger-feed him the cherries.

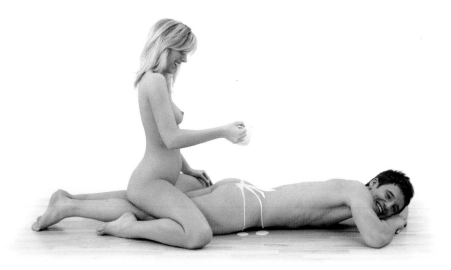

Drizzle cream over his buttocks, and lickable bits.

Perfect for: Giving him an after-dinner treat.
Irresistible when: You feverishly lap him up.

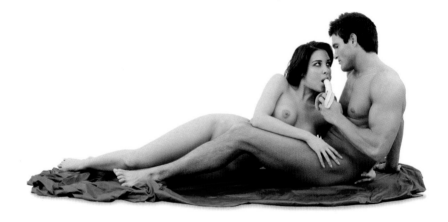

Slide your hot, soft lips as far down a banana as you can.

Perfect for: Not-in-the-least-bit-subtle symbolism.
Irresistible when: You use your lips on his fruity parts afterward.

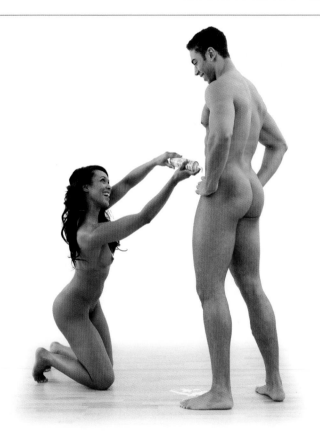

Fire aerosol whipped cream at his milk machine.

Perfect for: Delivering a fast blast of creamy pleasure.
Irresistible when: You ask if you can lick his Mr. Whippy.

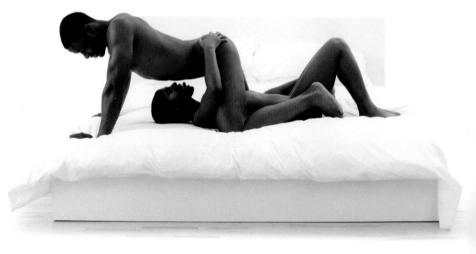

Slide underneath him, and flick your tongue in his belly button.

Perfect for: Giving him hot, deep thrumming in his engine room.
Irresistible when: You whisper "Lower, mate?"

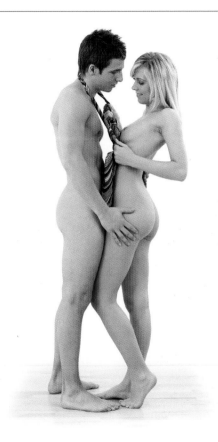

Grab the ends of his scarf, and pull him close.

Perfect for: The sheer delight of that "I've-been-captured" feeling.
Irresistible when: You reel him in for some warming lip action.

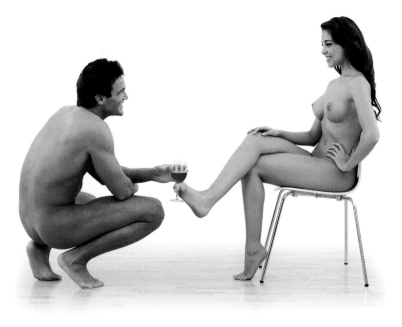

Let him sip wine from between your toes.

Perfect for: Playful frolics for guys with a thing about feet.
Irresistible when: You dip your toes in the wine, and he licks it off.

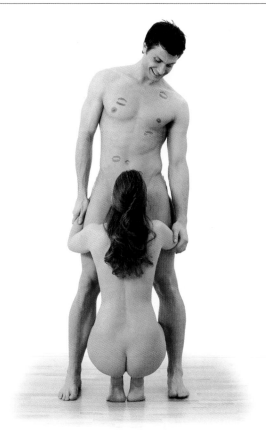

Leave crimson kisses on him from chest to crotch.

Perfect for: When he loves being marked by your gorgeous red lips.
Irresistible when: He looks on, as you paint his manhood.

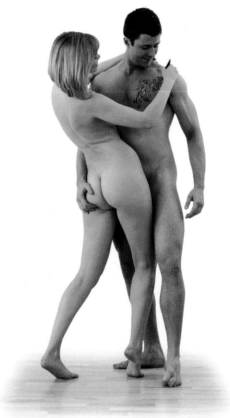

Get up close, and draw a sexy design on his chest with a body pen.

Perfect for: Giving him shivers as you swirl your nib on his skin.
Irresistible when: You take your pen south in a teasing, meandering line.

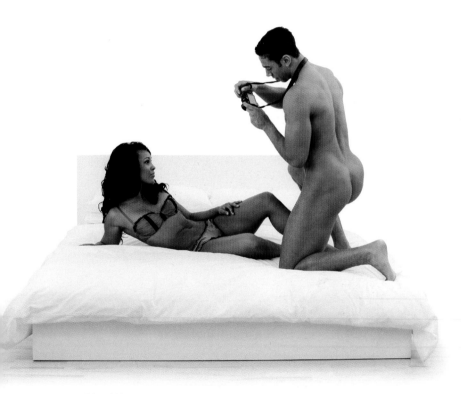

Hand him a camera, lie back, and make eyes at his lens.

Perfect for: Bringing your sexiest bits into sharp focus.
Irresistible when: You slip your bra off for maximum exposure.

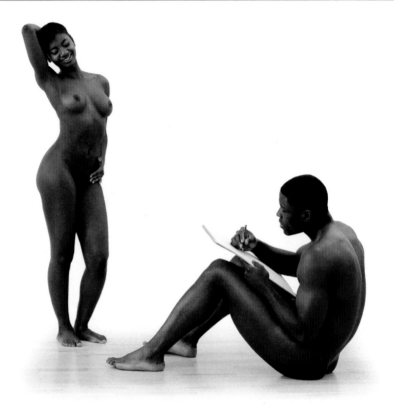

Strip off, strike a pose, then ask him to sketch you.

Perfect for: Giving him an artist's appreciation of your loveliness.
Irresistible when: His own penmanship gets him engorged.

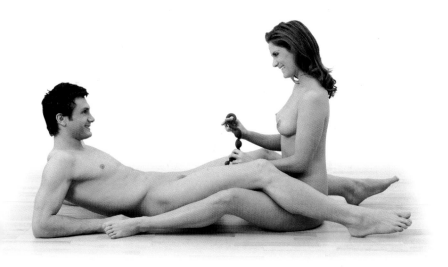

Gently insert some anal beads into his back buttonhole.

Perfect for: Pleasuring him with some exquisitely sensual penetration.
Irresistible when: You pull them out slowly at the moment of climax.

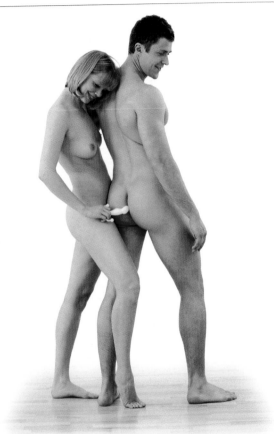

Insert a lubricated butt plug into him—getting him to bend over helps.

Perfect for: Opening his mind to the idea of P-spot bliss.
Irresistible when: He buffs his banana at the same time.

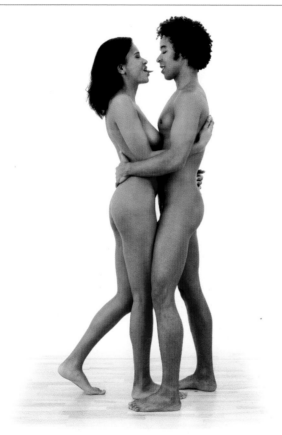

Poke your tongue out at him to reveal a tongue vibrator.

Perfect for: Less talk, more action.
Irresistible when: You slink down his body, and vibrate his frenulum.

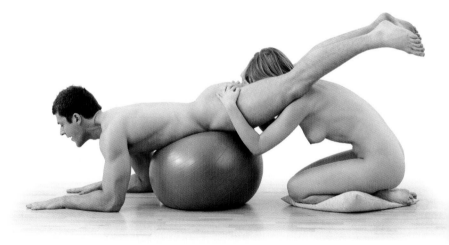

Interrupt his exercise routine to nestle your face between his legs.

Perfect for: Sending quivers down even the strongest of thighs.
Irresistible when: You give his man muscle a solid workout.

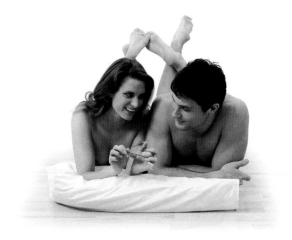

Get cozy, and tell him about your latest sex toy.

Perfect for: Getting him to say "Shall we?"
Irresistible when: You slip it on him during a sultry kiss.

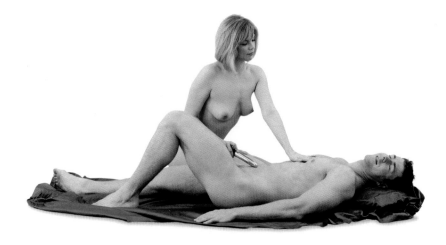

Whip out your vibrator, and draw patterns on his X-rated zones.

Perfect for: Giving him a delicious buzz in mind and body.
Irresistible when: You pop a boy-toy in his butt to really electrify him.

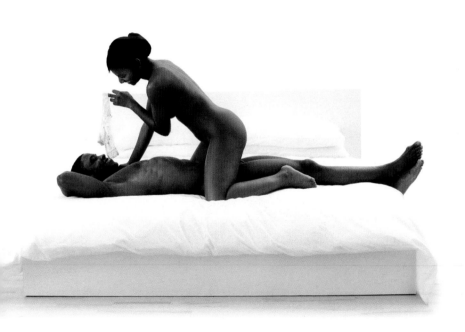

Whip your panties off and tickle his nose with them.

Perfect for: Giving him a ravenous appetite.
Irresistible when: You move up his body, and let him taste you at source.

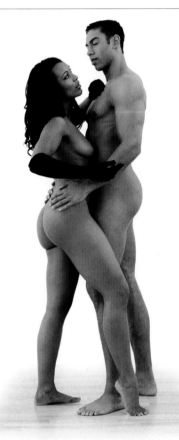

Pull on some elbow-length gloves, and cover his body with silky caresses.

Perfect for: A fizzing combination of elegance and sexual power.
Irresistible when: Coupled with a black bustier and fishnets.

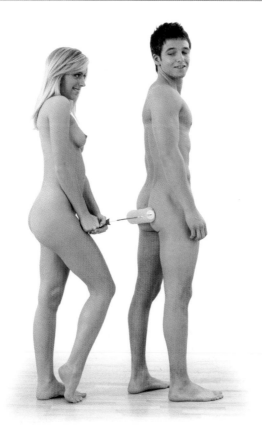

Roll a furry paint roller over his buttocks.

Perfect for: Treating him to a naughty night of bedroom DIY.
Irresistible when: You glide your roller over more of his hot contours.

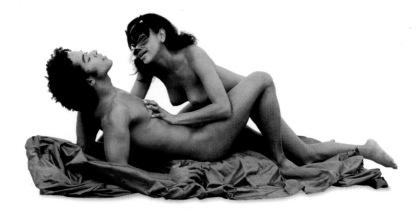

Play the part of his seductive sex kitten.

Perfect for: When he loves to be passionately scratched and clawed.
Irresistible when: You purr his name lustfully.

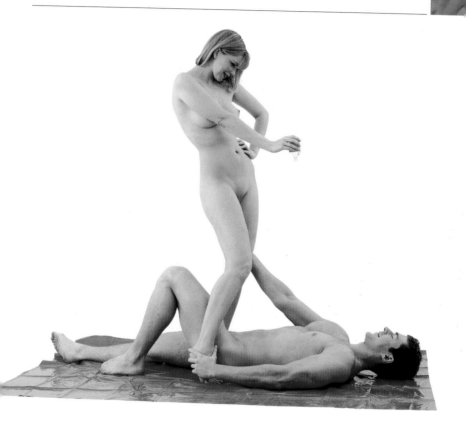

Lay him on a PVC sheet, and drizzle warm massage oil all over him.

Perfect for: When he's in need of a whole-body massage.
Irresistible when: You rub in the oil by slithering all over him voluptuously.

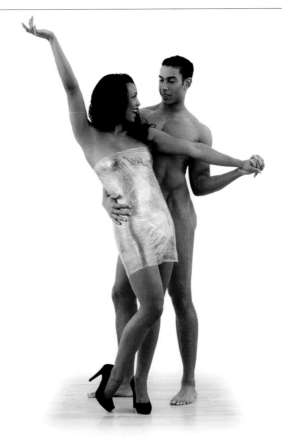

Get the kinky, see-through look—wear cling film.

Perfect for: Leaving nothing to his imagination.
Irresistible when: You spin around while he holds a corner of your dress.

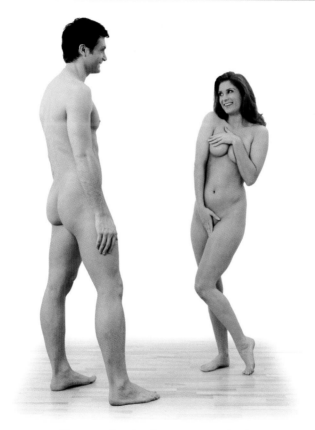

Play coy when he discovers you naked.

Perfect for: Sending a surprise rush of blood to his man zone.
Irresistible when: You hold back a little when he touches you.

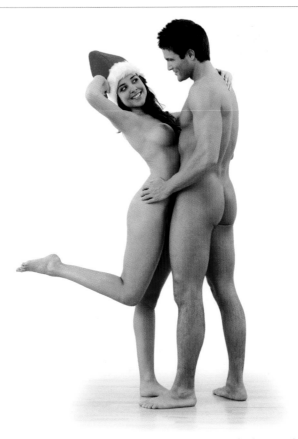

Put on your Santa hat, and make a gift of yourself.

Perfect for: Giving him a sweet ache in his baubles.
Irresistible when: You insist on basting his turkey with your tongue.

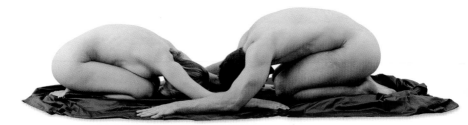

Teach him the Tantric ritual of bowing to a lover.

Perfect for: The ultimate gift of erotic surrender.
Irresistible when: You offer to be his eager-to-please Tantric goddess.

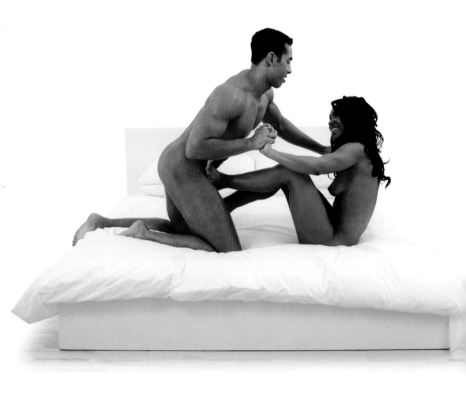

Pull him onto the bed for a romping and rolling play-fight.

Perfect for: Sitting on top of him, and holding him down.
Irresistible when: You tackle him with some hand-to-gland combat.

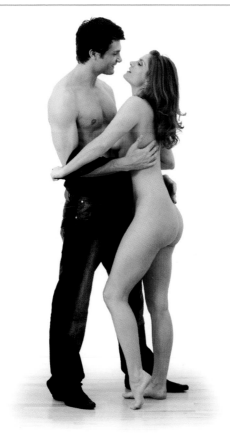

Lustfully rip off his shirt.

Perfect for: Setting him on fire with urgent passion.
Irresistible when: You fall to your knees, and tear his fly open.

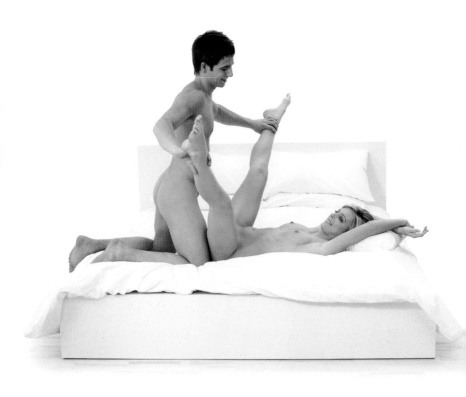

Invite him to help you with your early-morning power stretches.

Perfect for: Making his own muscle swell in the process.
Irresistible when: You catch his eye, and beckon him down for a teasing kiss.

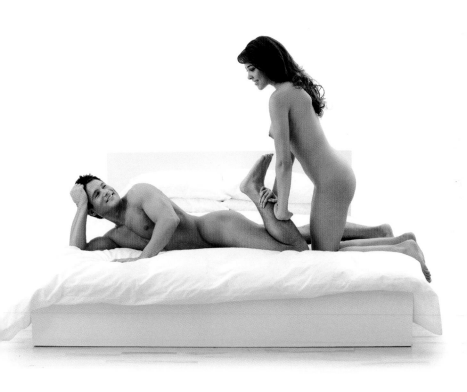

Pull, pummel, press, bend, knead, and rub his body until he feels like putty.

Perfect for: Putting him entirely at your mercy.
Irresistible when: You ask if he'd like a happy ending.

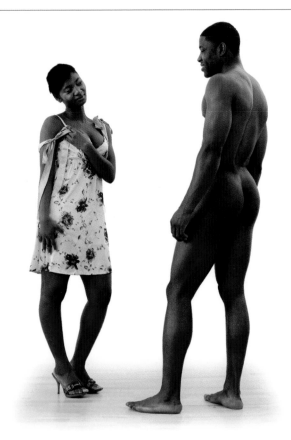

Tickle his fancy with a dress that keeps threatening to slip off.

Perfect for: Keeping his admiring gaze trained firmly on you.
Irresistible when: Oops, you accidentally lose your dress.

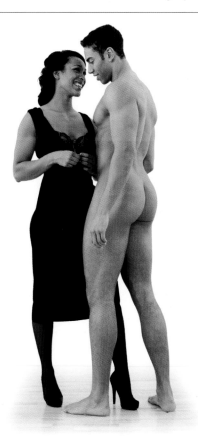

Take him somewhere private, undo some buttons, and put your cleavage on show.

Perfect for: Illicit encounters when he's in need of a treat.
Irresistible when: You ask him to slip his tongue between your breasts.

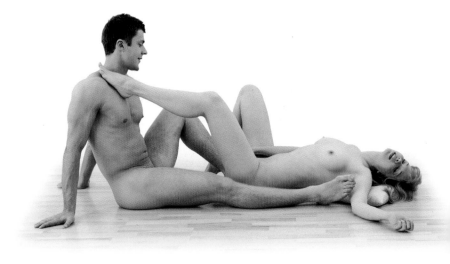

Give him a front-row seat while you pleasure yourself.

Perfect for: Live erotica right in front of his eyes.
Irresistible when: You tell him in a breathless gasp how badly you want him.

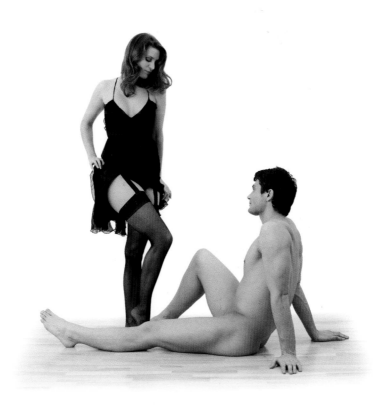

Give him a quick peek of what's under your dress just as you're leaving the house.

Perfect for: Encouraging him to pounce in public.
Irresistible when: You indulge in a steamy make-out session in the taxi home.

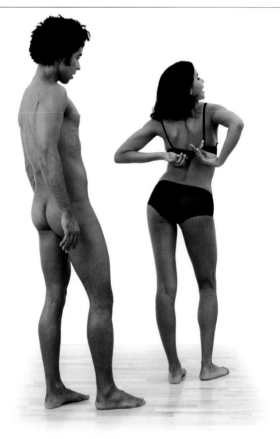

Unhook your bra in the final stages of a striptease.

Perfect for: Making him crave the delicious moment when you turn around.
Irresistible when: You're enjoying it as much as he is.

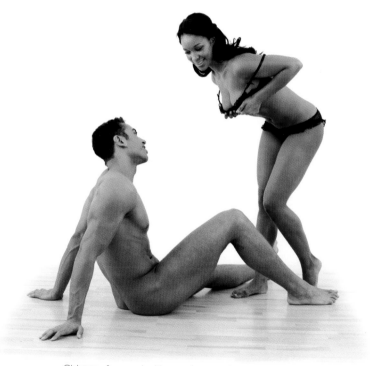

Shimmy forward with your breasts barely covered.

Perfect for: When he likes to be titillated burlesque-style.
Irresistible when: You whip off your bra to reveal naughty nipple tassels.

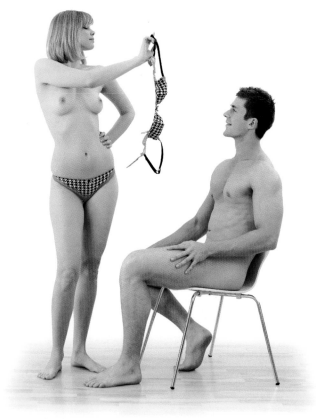

Reveal your body to him, one sexy bit at a time. Drop your bra into his lap.

Perfect for: Flirty and dirty weekends.
Irresistible when: You give him your panties as a souvenir.

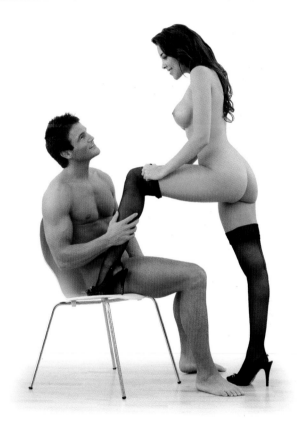

Rest your stocking-clad leg on his chair. Uncover your smooth-as-cream skin.

Perfect for: Making him feel as though his prayers have been answered.
Irresistible when: You sit astride him, and plant an angelic kiss on his lips.

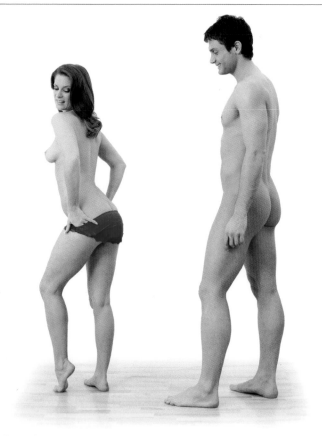

Bend forward slightly, and slide your panties down over your bottom.

Perfect for: Making his manhood bulge, and his blood run hot.
Irresistible when: You do it with delicious slowness.

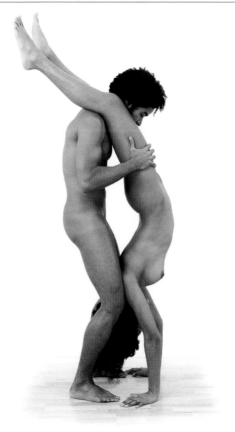

Ask him to catch your legs as you do a naked handstand.

Perfect for: Giving him a private peep show.
Irresistible when: You open your legs in a wide "v".

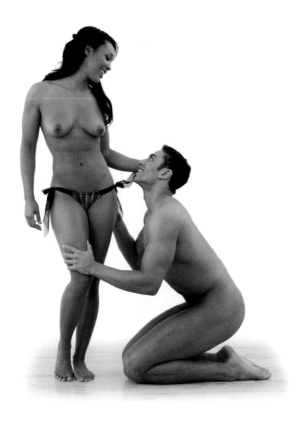

Put one of your ribbons in his mouth, and invite him to pull you.

Perfect for: Presenting him with a beautifully wrapped birthday gift.
Irresistible when: Your pubes are waxed into a heart shape.

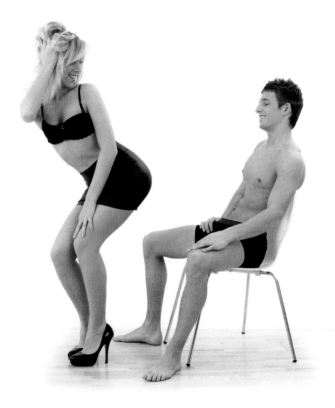

Bend over wearing a skirt that is barely wider than a belt.

Perfect for: Leaving him open-mouthed and passion-hungry.
Irresistible when: You let him take in the view, then ask to sit on his lap.

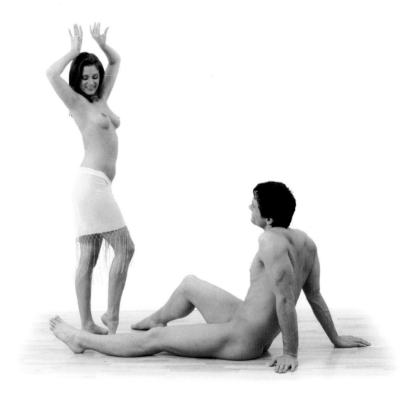

Perform a topless belly dance for him.

Perfect for: Hooking him with hot-from-the-harem sexiness.
Irresistible when: You get close to him, and flick your hips.

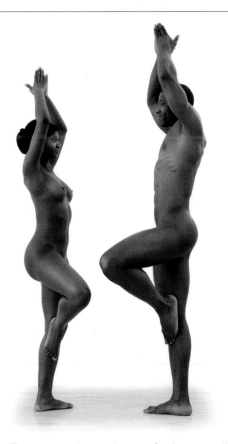

Play adult statues. The person who topples over first becomes the erotic servant.

Perfect for: Sex parties for two when the guests are well lubricated.
Irresistible when: You wobble, and put yourself at his service.

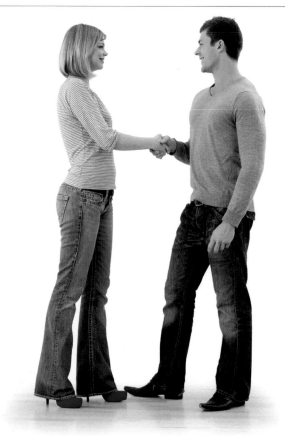

Introduce yourself as though you've never met—be flirty and bold.

Perfect for: Parties where no-one knows you're a couple.
Irresistible when: You say "Like to come back to my place for coffee?"

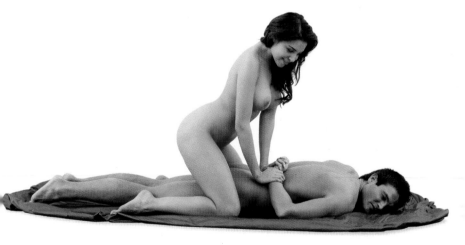

Pin him underneath you in a sexy straddle. Hold his wrists against his back.

Perfect for: Giving him deliciously nervous frissons about what's coming next.
Irresistible when: You devise a very bad plan. And you tell him about it.

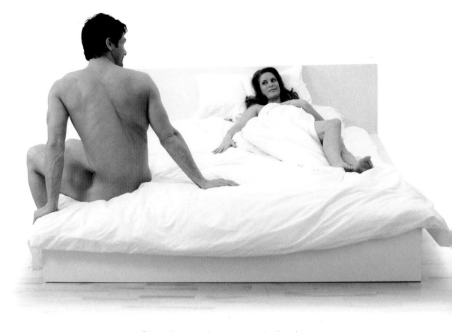

Give him your best come-to-bed eyes.

Perfect for: Making him feel like a sex god.
Irresistible when: You hold his gaze, and whip back the sheet.

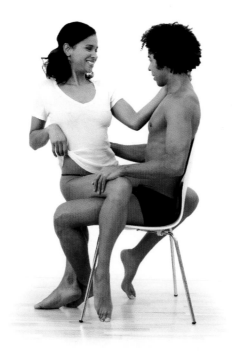

Seduce him by wearing a tight, wet T-shirt.

Perfect for: Making him feel like he'll explode if he doesn't get his hands on you.
Irresistible when: You press your cool, bare breasts against his burning body.

267 Naked worship

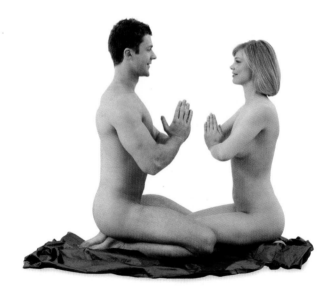

Honour him with a Tantric ritual—gaze into his eyes, and press your palms together.

Perfect for: Showering him with your divine love.
Irresistible when: You invite him into your inner sex sanctum.

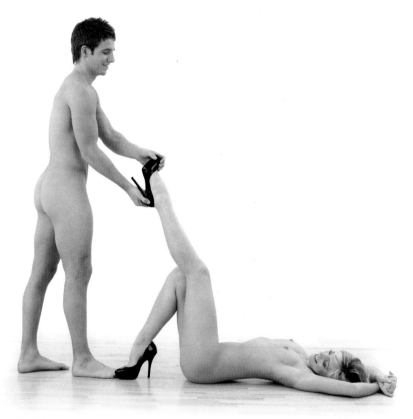

Stretch your legs in the air one at a time, and ask him to remove your killer heels.

Perfect for: Taking him to near-delirium at a very private, foot-fetish party.
Irresistible when: You wear your sexiest stockings and garter belt.

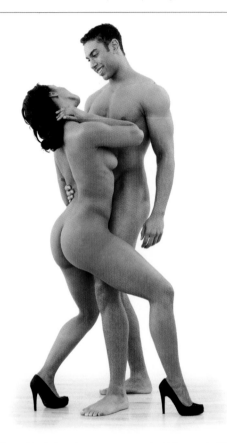

Seduce him with red-hot dancing—press against him, and slither down his body.

Perfect for: The raunchiest behavior you can get away with in public.
Irresistible when: You shimmy down his body with your back to him.

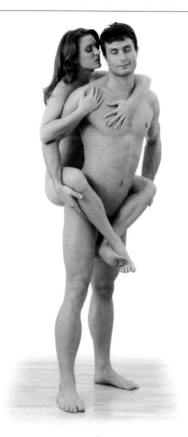

Whisper something filthy in his ear as you hitch a ride to the bedroom.

Perfect for: Giving him a delicious erotic chafing with your heels.
Irresistible when: Your hands go to work on his chest and nipples.

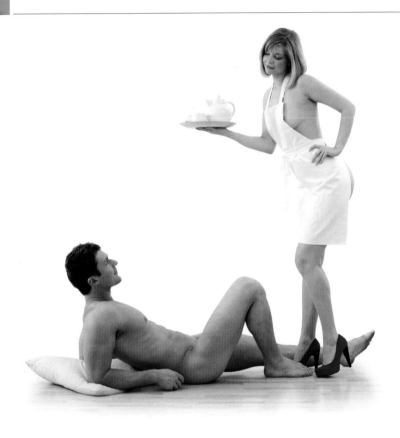

Dress in a crisp, white apron, and serve him tea with polite formality.

Perfect for: When decorum turns him on.
Irresistible when: You walk away with a wiggle of your bare butt.

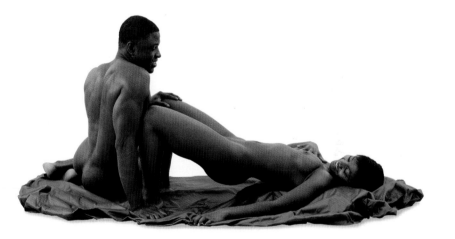

Pick your best provocative yoga posture, and go flaunt yourself.

Perfect for: Uncoiling his kundalini.
Irresistible when: You practice deep breathing at the same time.

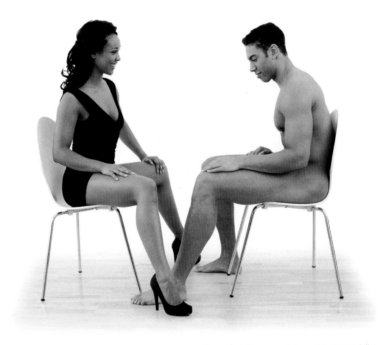

Cross and uncross your legs Sharon Stone-style – pantyless and in public.

Perfect for: Making him double up with desire.
Irresistible when: You smile wickedly as you prolong the torture.

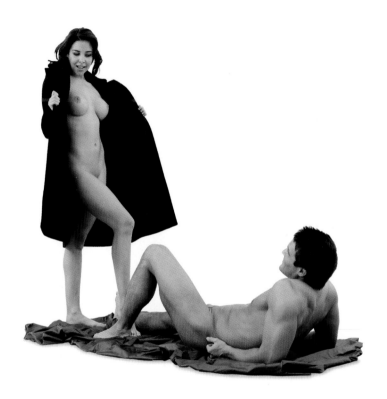

Whip your coat open wide to reveal—nada.

Perfect for: Taking him from 0–60 in a flash.
Irresistible when: You look him in the eye, and shimmy off your coat.

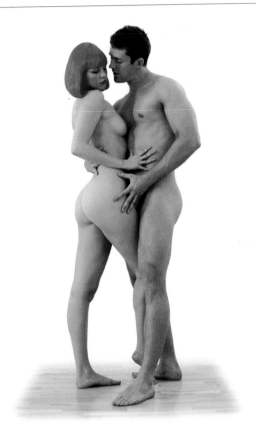

Put on a red wig and lipstick, and surprise him with your brazen behavior.

Perfect for: Bringing all his debauched fantasies about redheads to life.
Irresistible when: You play her fierce and fiery.

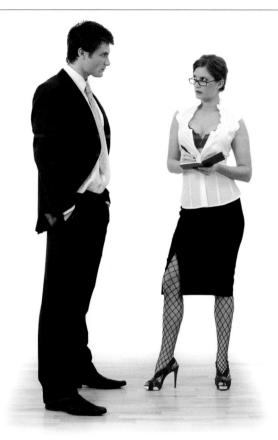

You're the sexy secretary. He's your strict boss. Play your role to the max.

Perfect for: When calling him "Sir" powers up his libido.
Irresistible when: You let your hair down, and take off your glasses.

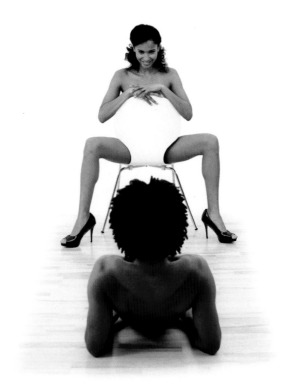

Take off all your clothes, and tease him by straddling a chair.

Perfect for: A photograph for his private, erotic album.
Irresistible when: You wink and beckon him toward you.

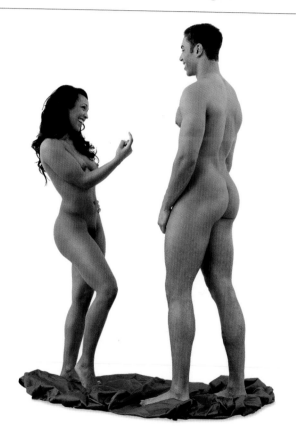

Throw him your sexiest look, and beckon him over.

Perfect for: When he gets off on stranger roleplay.
Irresistible when: You pull him onto the bed, and service him.

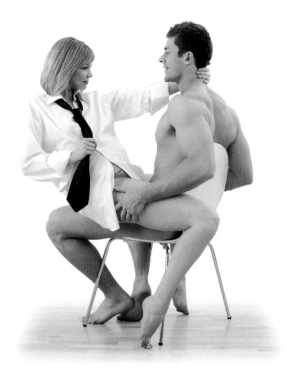

Slip into an oversize shirt and tie, then sidle sexily onto his lap.

Perfect for: When he lusts after girls, who look like office boys.
Irresistible when: You pop between his legs, and lay on some executive relief.

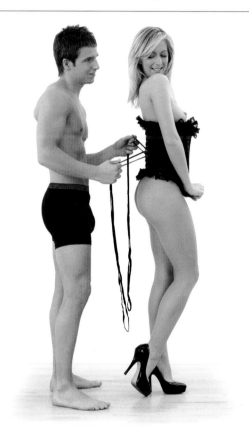

Ask him to free you from an ever-so-tight corset.

Perfect for: Inching up his arousal levels.
Irresistible when: You turn around naked with a wicked glint in your eye.

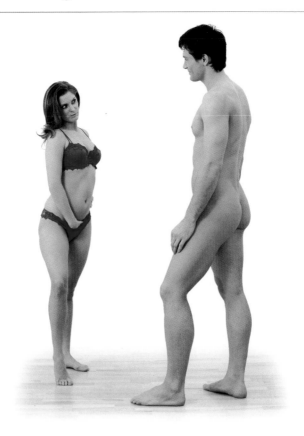

Slide your hands into your panties while he watches.

Perfect for: Giving him voyeuristic thrills.
Irresistible when: You multitask by stroking his treasures too.

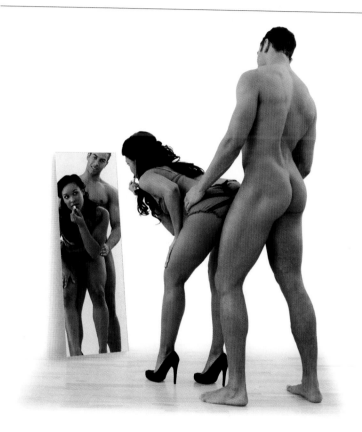

Catch his eye in the mirror with a provocative look as you put your lipstick on.

Perfect for: Filling him with taut, sexual tension.
Irresistible when: You wink naughtily, and blow him a kiss.

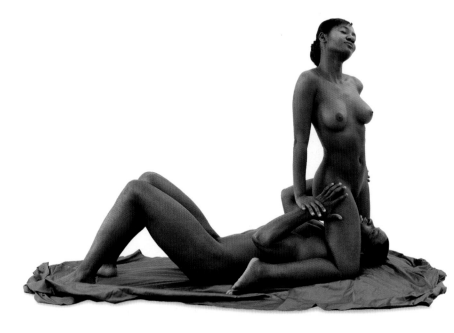

Tantalize him by kneeling over his face, and circling your hips s-l-o-w-l-y.

Perfect for: The sweet pain of being so-near-yet-so-far.
Irresistible when: You slide your fingers inside your palace gates.

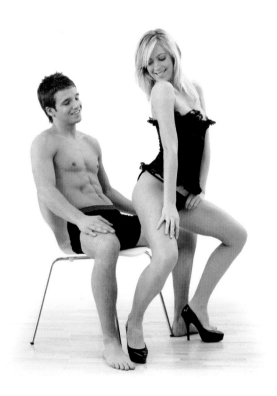

Stick your ass out, turn out your feet, and circle your hips.

Perfect for: Getting him rock-hard and ready.
Irresistible when: You throw a coy glance at him over your shoulder.

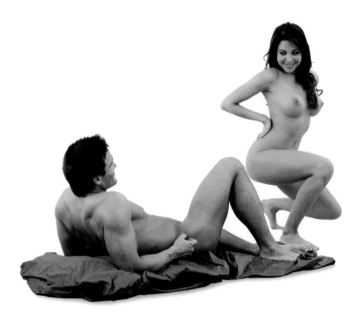

Arch your back, stick your chest out, and circle your pelvis. Now, bend your knees.

Perfect for: Making him hungry with longing.
Irresistible when: You do it while standing astride him.

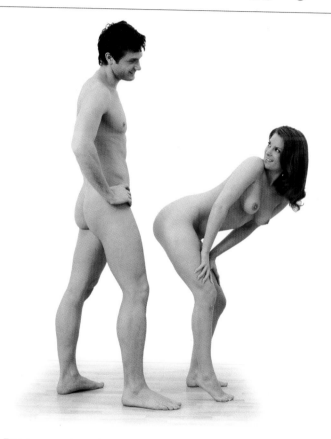

Bend over, put your hands on your knees, and wiggle your bottom.

Perfect for: Making his day.
Irresistible when: You wriggle up close, so your peaches nudge his plums.

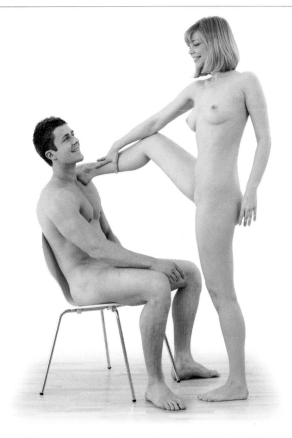

Show off your suppleness by pressing your foot against his shoulder.

Perfect for: A close-up that makes him throb.
Irresistible when: You run your hand from calf to thigh with seductive slowness.

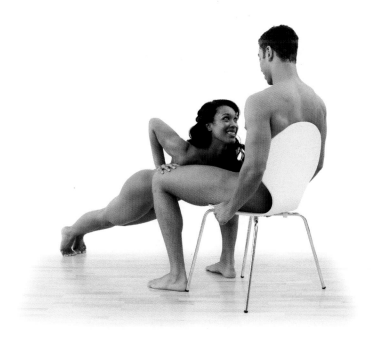

Use him as your workout bench—start with push-ups.

Perfect for: The joy of seeing you bobbing up and down in his lap.
Irresistible when: Your face lands tongue-distance from his package.

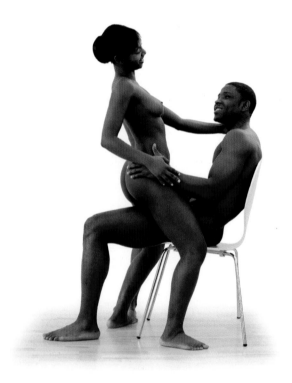

Perform the lap-dancing trick of riding his thigh without touching it.

Perfect for: A fast way to trigger his erotic lust.
Irresistible when: You accidently brush him, and he feels your forbidden juices.

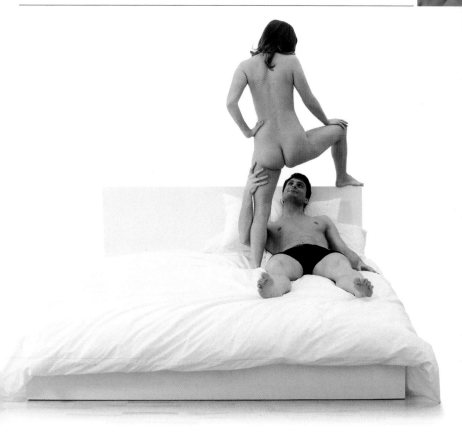

Strike a pose by standing above him with one leg raised.

Perfect for: Giving him intoxicating, porn-style close-ups.
Irresistible when: You make it the climax of a striptease.

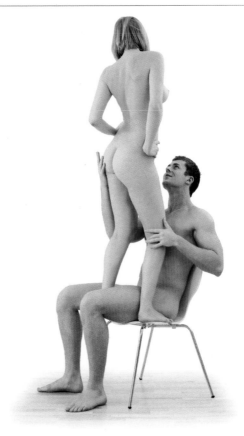

Try this advanced lap-dancing move—circle your hips while standing astride him.

Perfect for: Giving him weeks of fantasy fodder.
Irresistible when: You lean over, and graze his lips with your nipples.

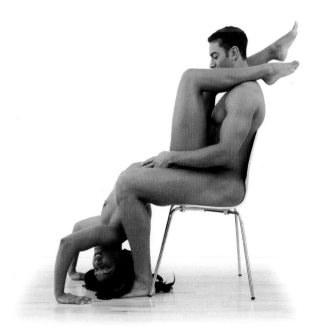

Show off your sexpertise—make this move the climax of a lap dance.

Perfect for: Making him wonder why he ever leaves the house.
Irresistible when: You can do the splits upside-down too.

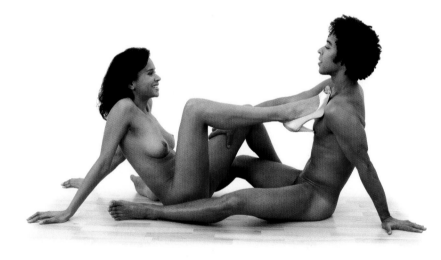

Gently press your stiletto heel into his chest.

Perfect for: Giving him spiky thrills.
Irresistible when: You slide both feet onto his shoulders, and lie back.

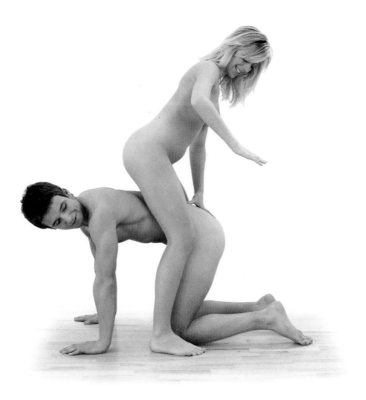

Order him to his knees, and spank him squarely on the butt.

Perfect for: When rough handling makes him rampantly horny.
Irresistible when: You act like you mean it.

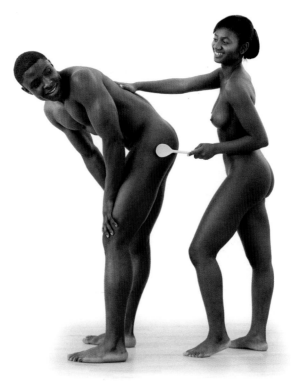

Whack him with a wooden spoon when he's misbehaving.

Perfect for: Rampant kinkiness in the kitchen.
Irresistible when: You grease his body with butter, and pounce.

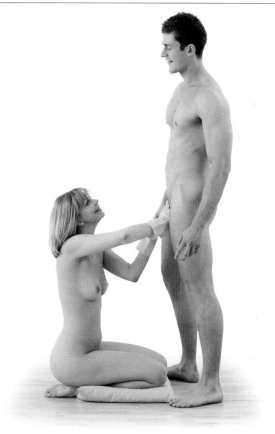

Pop on a pair of rubber gloves, and give him a handjob.

Perfect for: When rubber caresses take him straight to paradise.
Irresistible when: Your gloves are hot, wet, and slick with lube.

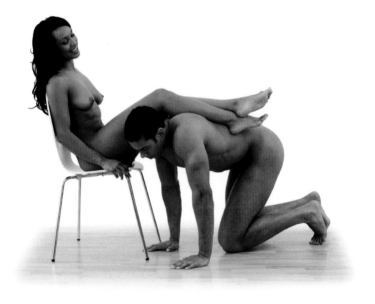

Have a dominatrix day—order him to be your foot soldier.

Perfect for: When treating him mean makes him super-keen.
Irresistible when: You have a list of degrading jobs to make him pant for more.

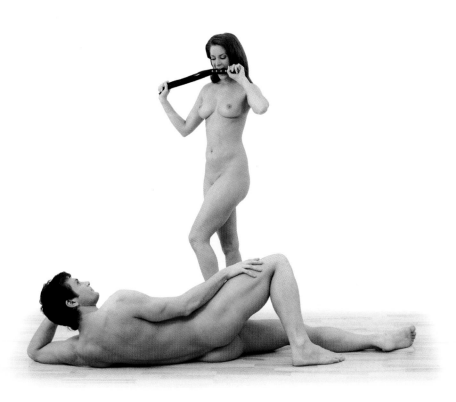

Show him your mean side—brandish a strap or whip.

Perfect for: Guys with a penchant for pain.
Irresistible when: You tie him to the bedposts, and tell him there is no escape.

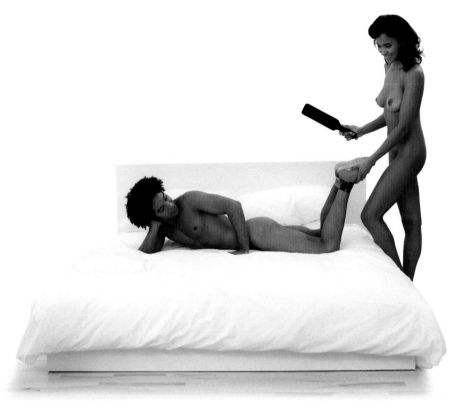

Bind his ankles with bondage tape, and pat his soles with a paddle.

Perfect for: Blissful tingles that surge through him.
Irresistible when: You alternate the taps with sole-ful kisses.

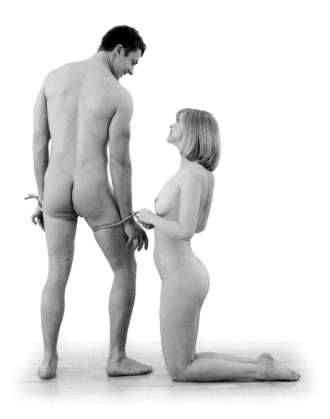

Trap his hands against his thighs using kinky spank ties.

Perfect for: Giving him a stiffy of steel as you cavort in front of him.
Irresistible when: You wrap your lips around his rod.

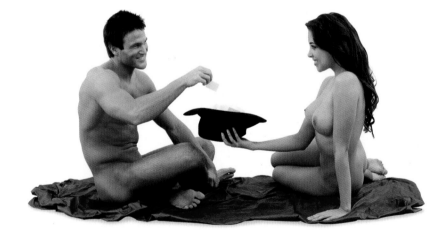

Fill a hat with kinky dares, and ask him to pull one out.

Perfect for: Giving him an excuse to do something filthy to you.
Irresistible when: You're game for absolutely anything too.

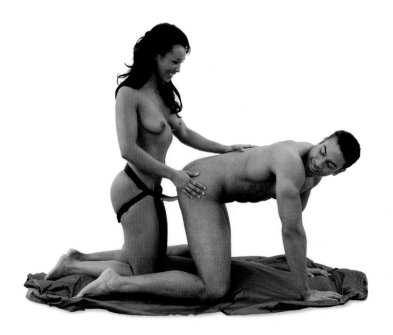

Strap yourself into a kinky leather harness complete with dildo.

Perfect for: Making sparks fly in his private erotic chamber.
Irresistible when: You swirl your lubed tip softly on his perimeter.

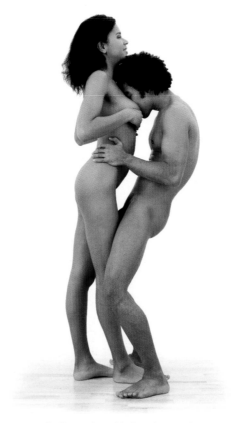

231 Bosom pals

Softly enclose his face in your breasts.

Perfect for: When he can't take his eyes off your cleavage.
Irresistible when: You repeat the embrace on his broom handle.

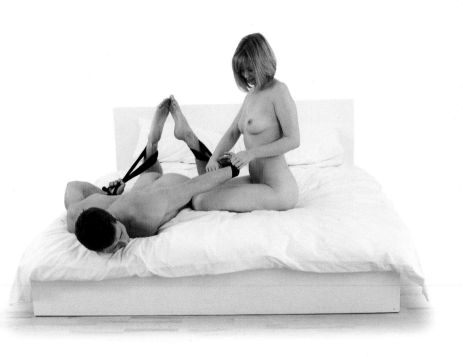

Be wicked—strap his ankles to his wrists, and take advantage of him.

Perfect for: Making him moan with erotic frustration.
Irresistible when: You massage his body with your breasts.

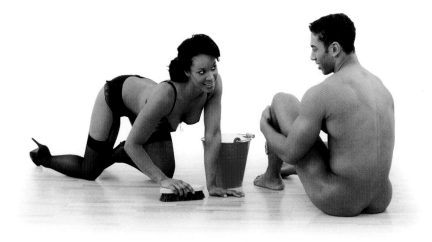

Show your servility by scrubbing the floor in heels and underwear.

Perfect for: When sexy submission drives him insane with desire.
Irresistible when: You crawl close, and ask him in a whisper for your next task.

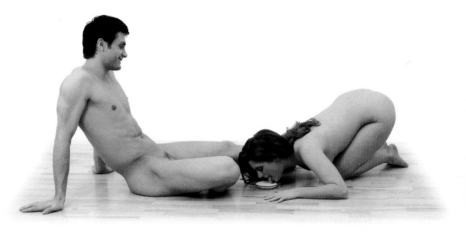

Lick cream from a bowl as you play the part of his submissive sex kitten.

Perfect for: Making him hard with the sight of your soft, strokable skin.
Irresistible when: You slink toward him with a dirty look in your eye.

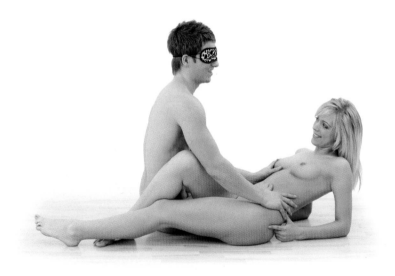

Blindfold him, then offer him your naked body.

Perfect for: The naughty delight of exploring any bit he likes.
Irresistible when: You part your legs to welcome his hands.

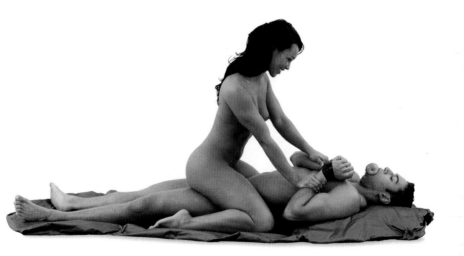

Commence his slave training—bind his wrists and "gag" him with an apple.

Perfect for: When enforced vulnerability makes him super-horny.
Irresistible when: You dress in tight, black PVC.

225 Lewd limbo

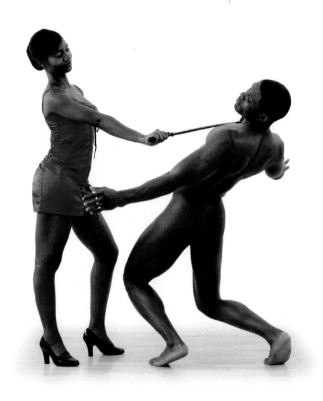

Tell him you'll take your dress off, if he makes it under your cane.

Perfect for: The thrill of being forced to earn his sexual treats.
Irresistible when: The harder his erection, the firmer your discipline.

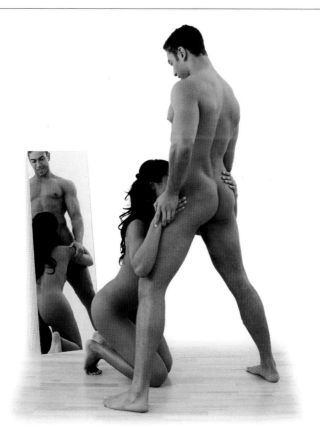

Slide your lips up and down his member while he watches from two directions.

Perfect for: Making him feel like he's part of a porn film.
Irresistible when: You do it side on to the mirror for maximum erotic impact.

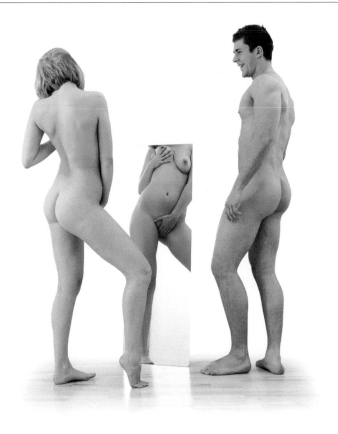

Pretend you're alone as you caress yourself in front of a mirror.

Perfect for: Giving him illicit, peep-show pleasures.
Irresistible when: You forget he's there, and get carried away.

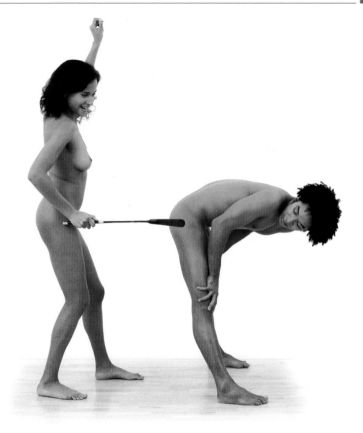

Tell him to bend over, then thwack him with your riding crop.

Perfect for: When he's desperate to be ridden by you.
Irresistible when: You lay him on the ground, and mount him seductively.

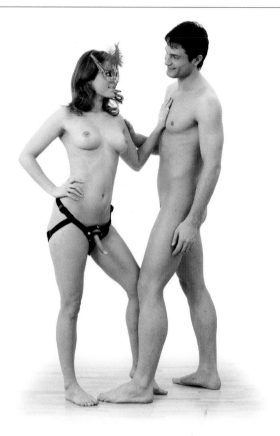

Throw a private kink party for him.

Perfect for: Indulging his fantasies, and making him feel like a very bad boy.
Irresistible when: You lay him on his front, then slide provocatively onto his back.

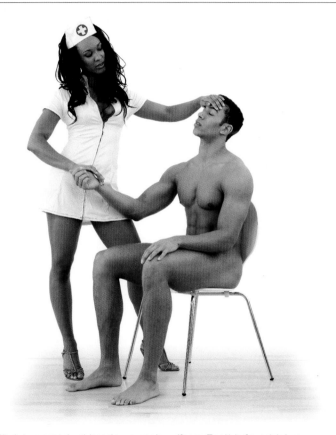

Slip into a crotch-skimming nurse's uniform. Feel his feverish brow.

Perfect for: Putting him in a safe and sexy pair of hands.
Irresistible when: You offer to examine that hard swelling in his lap.

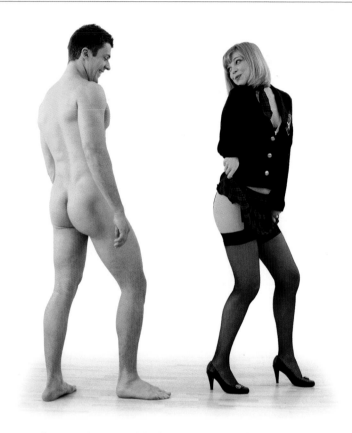

Squeeze into your old school uniform, and flirt outrageously.

Perfect for: Reliving the horny ecstasy of schoolboy crushes.
Irresistible when: You ask for help with your homework—in bed.

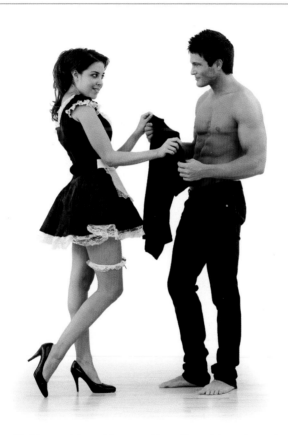

Be his naughty maid—serve him with a wink and a pout.

Perfect for: Making him feel like the beddable master.
Irresistible when: You know what he wants before he does.

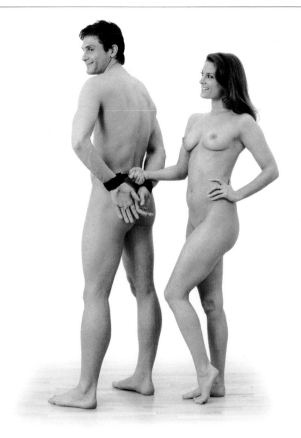

Grab him playfully, and tie his wrists together behind his back.

Perfect for: Guys who like girls to call the shots.
Irresistible when: You don't release him until he's delirious with desire.

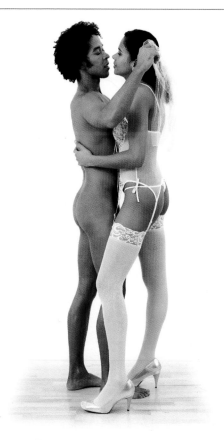

Play the virginal bride dying to be taken.

Perfect for: Letting him honor your offer the way he likes best.
Irresistible when: You take it s-l-o-w-l-y.

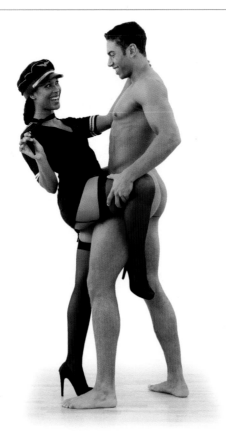

Introduce yourself as his flirty flight attendant—"I'll be looking after you tonight".

Perfect for: Putting his engines on full-throttle.
Irresistible when: You strip as part of the in-flight entertainment.

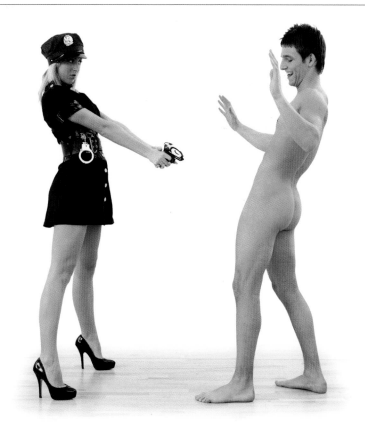

Play the bad, lady cop—point a water pistol at his package.

Perfect for: Guys who fantasize about being stripped and searched.
Irresistible when: Your pistol fires warm massage oil.

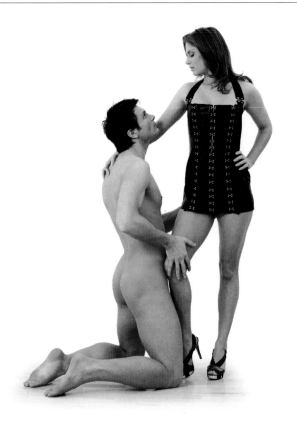

Dress in kinky leather, PVC, or rubber, and demand to be caressed.

Perfect for: When fetish-wear makes him weak and feverish.
Irresistible when: You're pantyless.

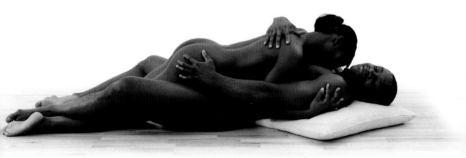

Be his sexy blanket—cover his bits with yours.

Perfect for: Giving his hands license to roam freely.
Irresistible when: You smother his chest with hungry kisses.

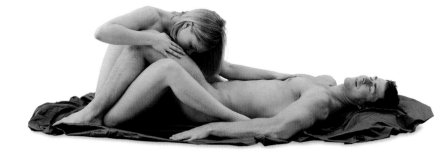

Lick, suck, nuzzle, and kiss your way up the inside of his leg.

Perfect for: Turning his loins to molten lava.
Irresistible when: Your hair happens to tickle and caress his twins.

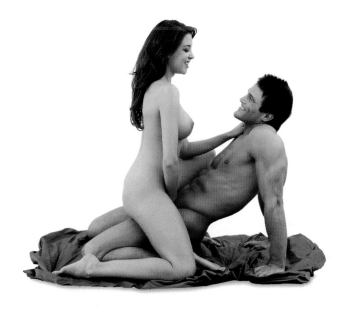

Sit astride him, and jiggle his peak against your crevice.

Perfect for: Taking him to dizzying heights of ecstasy.
Irresistible when: You pull him back when he's close to the summit.

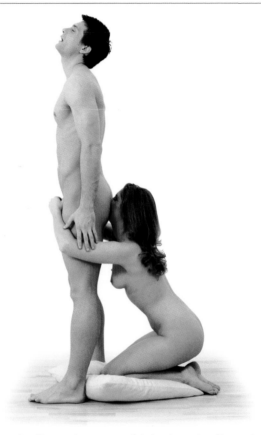

Tickle his back porch with your tongue, and his front porch with your hand.

Perfect for: Making his knees tremble.
Irresistible when: You get into climax-triggering rhythm.

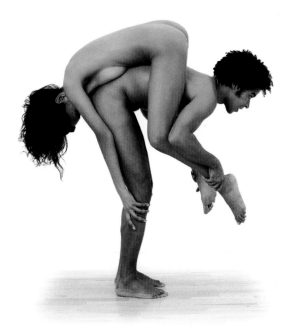

Balance on his back for a novel approach to anilingus.

Perfect for: Giving him a red-hot bolt of eroticism.
Irresistible when: You have a tongue with a long reach.

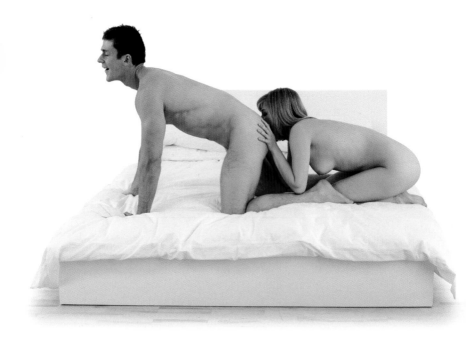

Kneel behind him, and practice your anilingus skills.

Perfect for: Introducing him to the raptures of rimming.
Irresistible when: Accompanied by light, fingertip caresses on his balls.

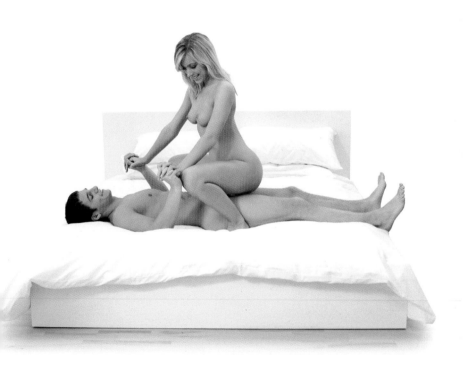

Do a deep squat, and tickle his bits with yours.

Perfect for: Teasing him remorselessly.
Irresistible when: Your thighs finally give way, and you sink onto him.

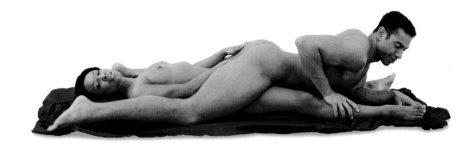

Press your lubed fingers along his cracks and crevices.

Perfect for: Velvety rear sensations, while his penis nestles between your thighs.
Irresistible when: Your fingers make a soft but deep rear entry.

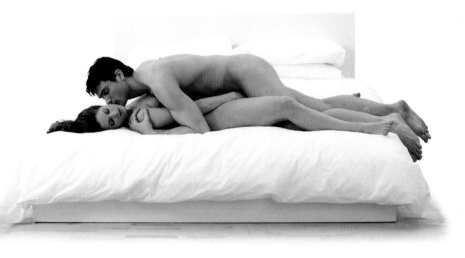

Reach down, and moisten his milkman by rubbing it against you.

Perfect for: Letting him know that you could rock his world at any second.
Irresistible when: You tantalize him by letting him almost slip inside.

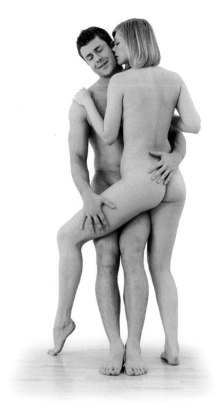

Press him against a wall, and slide your honeypot along his thigh.

Perfect for: Making him incoherent with desire.
Irresistible when: Your breath is fast, hot, and urgent in his ear.

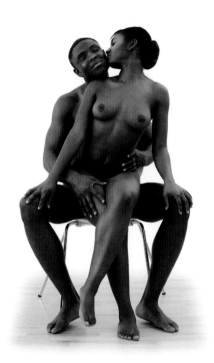

Slink onto his lap, and slide your tush against his package.

Perfect for: Luring him away from the TV or computer.
Irresistible when: You keep wiggling until you find a comfortable spot.

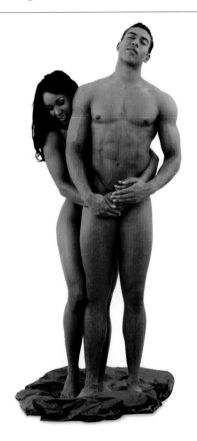

Stand behind him, and take him firmly in hand.

Perfect for: Simulating the juice-inducing strokes he'd use on himself.
Irresistible when: Your wrists work like a dynamo.

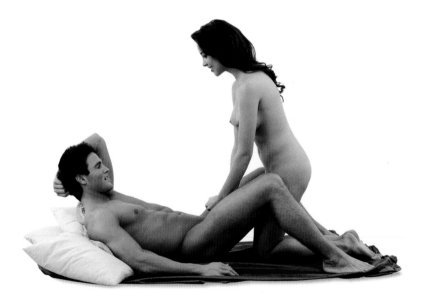

Kneel between his legs, and grab his gear shift.

Perfect for: Up-and-down strokes that are guaranteed to rev his engine.
Irresistible when: You drive him fast and furiously.

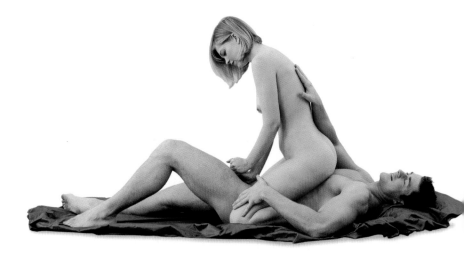

Straddle his chest, then curve your palms around his pole.

Perfect for: Smooth hand-over-hand slickness that makes him moan.
Irresistible when: You bend forward, so he can feast his eyes on your curves.

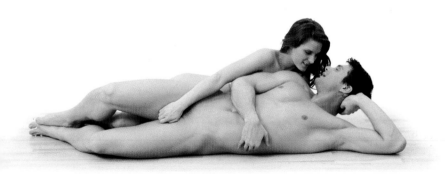

Reach down to caress his package while you're chatting.

Perfect for: Slow fondling that quickly gets steamy and intense.
Irresistible when: Your oiled hand pumps him until he's rigid with desire.

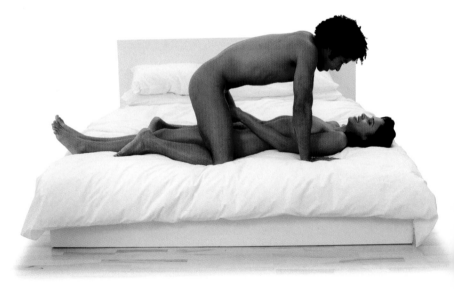

Stroke his shaft as he kneels over you.

Perfect for: The sexy thrill of being seduced back into bed.
Irresistible when: You juice him by swirling your fingertips on his tip.

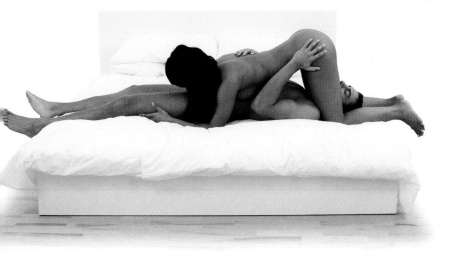

Drive him wild with a nearly-but-not-quite 69.

Perfect for: Letting him gaze longingly at the scenery.
Irresistible when: You slip for a moment, and make his face moist.

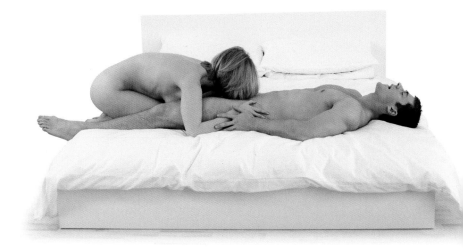

Give him a blowjob as he stretches out in comfort.

Perfect for: When he needs his powerful erection quickly soothed.
Irresistible when: You drive him wild by teasing his testicles with your tongue.

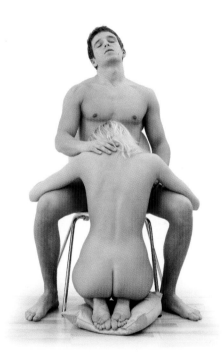

Kneel between his legs, and charm him with your expert tongue.

Perfect for: Seducing him at his desk after office hours.
Irresistible when: You stay down there for the duration.

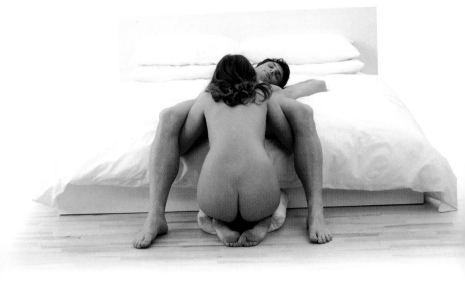

Kneel between his legs, and glide your lips wetly up and down his shaft.

Perfect for: Giving him an electric start to the day.
Irresistible when: You press the sexstasy spot on his perineum.

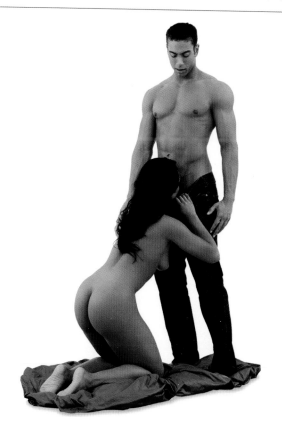

Unbutton his fly, and see what comes up.

Perfect for: When he requires an urgent seeing to.
Irresistible when: You're not afraid to tackle the root of the issue.

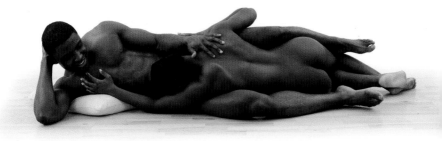

Be his favorite fellatrice—scoff him while he's lying on his side.

Perfect for: Interrupting a cuddle to dive under the covers.
Irresistible when: You grasp his buttocks, and pull him hard into your mouth.

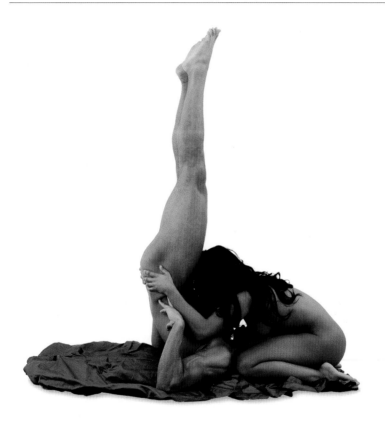

Get him to do a shoulder stand, then wrap your fiery mouth around his shuttle.

Perfect for: Sending him into sensual orbit.
Irresistible when: You deliver a performance worthy of Cape Canaveral.

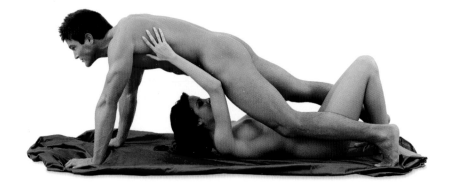

Lie open-mouthed below him while he does push-ups.

Perfect for: Letting him set a stimulating pace.
Irresistible when: You give your tongue muscles a thorough stretching.

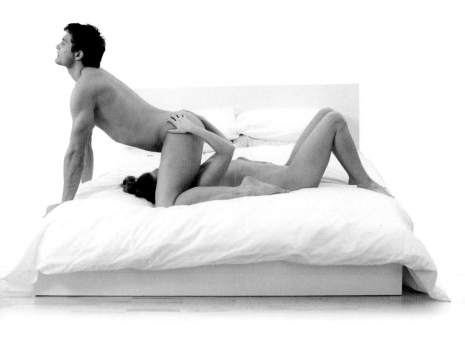

Pay him lip service from underneath while he's down on all fours.

Perfect for: The euphoria of being sexually served.
Irresistible when: You lick his underside with slavish devotion.

Polishing his pole

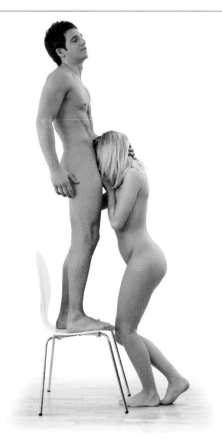

Lure him onto a chair, and slide your lips along his shaft.

Perfect for: Giving him an instant erotic high.
Irresistible when: You cup his balls in your hand, and swallow him whole.

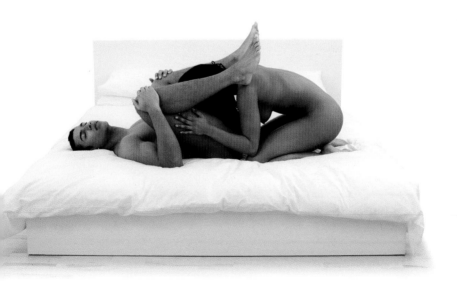

Pull his shaft back through his thighs, and agitate him with your tongue.

Perfect for: Making his rod glow red hot.
Irresistible when: You make him hover at the point of no return.

185 Swallowing him up

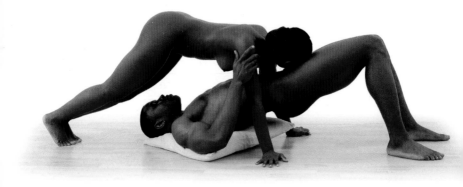

Meet him halfway as he raises his manhood to your lips.

Perfect for: Giving him some lust-enhancing visuals.
Irresistible when: You open wide, and get your tonsils tickled.

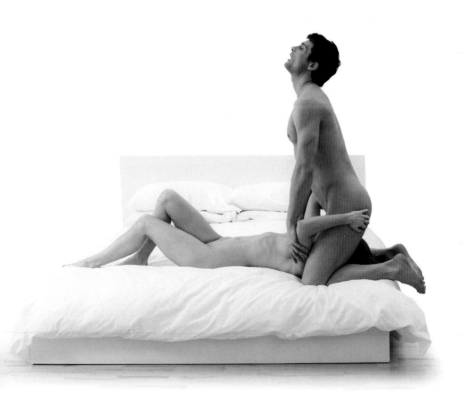

Caress his balls and perineum with your lips and tongue.

Perfect for: Intense undercarriage pleasure.
Irresistible when: He joins in, and strokes his package by hand.

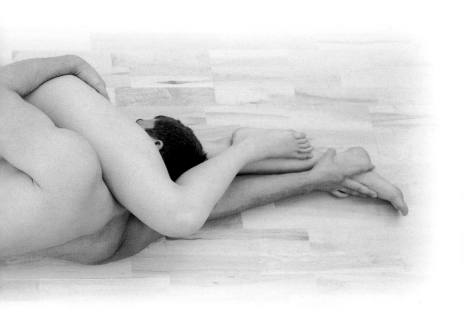

183 Do, as you would be done by

Lie top-to-tail, and take him in your mouth.

Perfect for: Setting up a pleasure circuit that will drive him wild.

Irresistible when: You lick and suck with frenzied abandon.

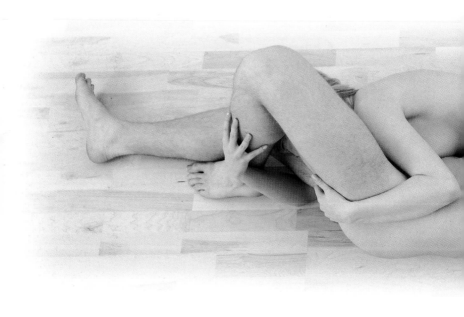

Lie top-to-tail, and push your head between her thighs.

Perfect for: When giving and receiving is her path to ecstasy.
Irresistible when: You keep your head tightly in the game.

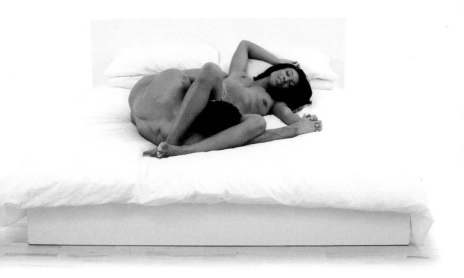

Wriggle your head between her legs, and make leisurely lip-love to her.

Perfect for: Taking a slow but sublimely seductive approach.
Irresistible when: You're happy to lie there all day long.

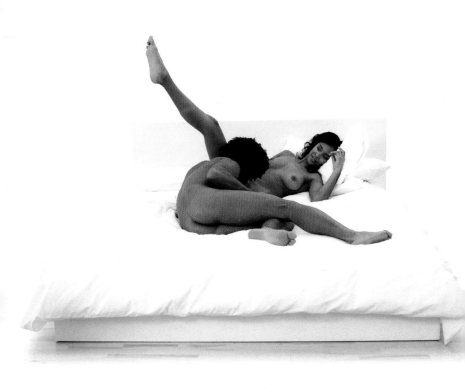

181 Giving her a leg up

Nuzzle her carnal cave as she rests her leg on your shoulder.

Perfect for: Finding her hidden treasures with your tongue.
Irresistible when: You shake your head in situ as though saying "No".

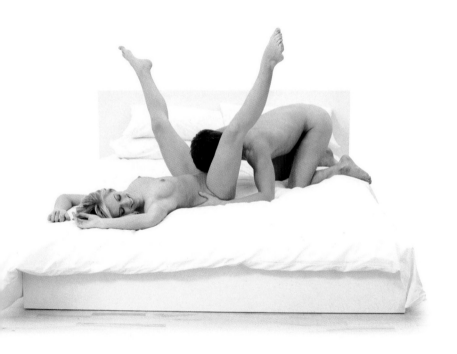

Bury your face between her thighs as she opens her legs in a sexy "V".

Perfect for: Making her feel utterly adored on your anniversary.
Irresistible when: You go down with a smile on your face.

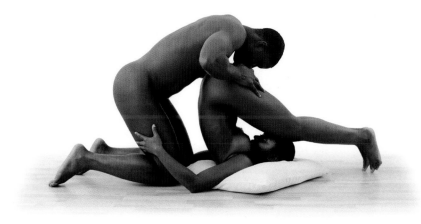

Put her feet behind her head, then apply your special lip balm.

Perfect for: Curing the ache between her legs.
Irresistible when: You kiss her better by whirling your tongue.

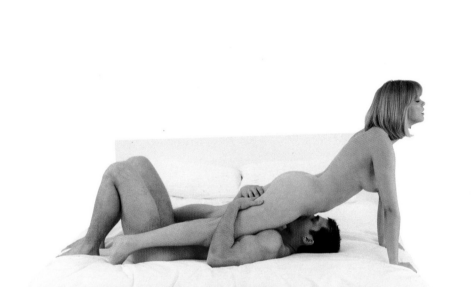

Twirl your tongue on her while she's in a push-up position.

Perfect for: Making trembles of pleasure course through her body.
Irresistible when: You pulse your tongue on her until she can't take any more.

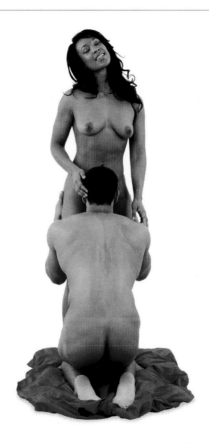

Hold her hips in your hands, and demand entry with your tongue.

Perfect for: The sudden excitement of an unexpected guest.
Irresistible when: You repeatedly jab her joy buzzer.

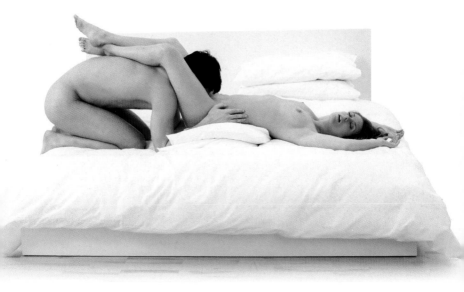

Raise her hips on some pillows, then go in search of her pearl.

Perfect for: Getting comfortable, and taking her oral pleasure seriously.
Irresistible when: You tease out her pearl, and suck very gently.

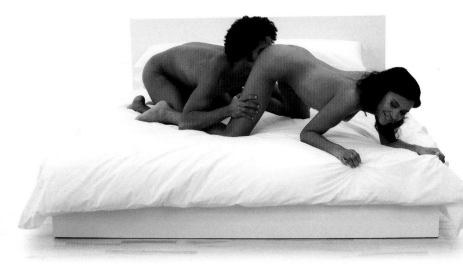

Give her a tongue bath while she kneels on all fours.

Perfect for: Giving her vulnerable, yet very naughty, feelings.
Irresistible when: You lick her with a soft and yielding tongue.

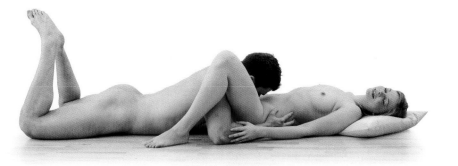

Part her legs, then let your tongue weave its magic.

Perfect for: Swirling, licking, and nuzzling that takes her breath away.
Irresistible when: Moans of ecstasy escape from your lips.

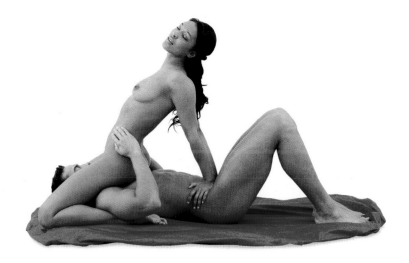

Invite her to straddle your face while you devour her.

Perfect for: Giving her the freedom to rock, roll, slip, and slide.
Irresistible when: You help her to gyrate with your hands on her hips.

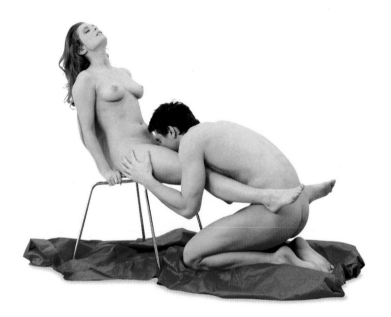

Sit her down, and worship her with your tongue.

Perfect for: When she wants to look down from above.
Irresistible when: You use your fingers too, and get a spirited rhythm going.

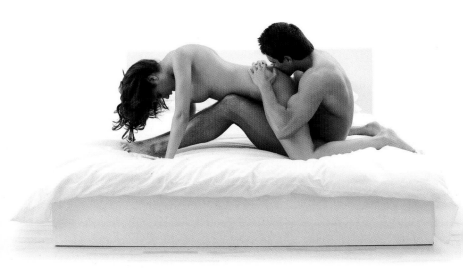

Support her with your knees as you circle her rear star with your tongue.

Perfect for: Transporting her to a distant planet of bliss.
Irresistible when: You use your tongue like a probe.

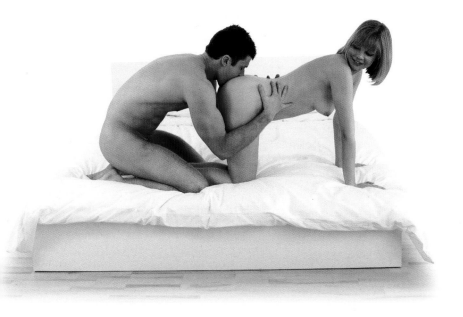

Caress her anus with your tongue.

Perfect for: Making her blossom with desire.
Irresistible when: You follow up with some focused green-fingering.

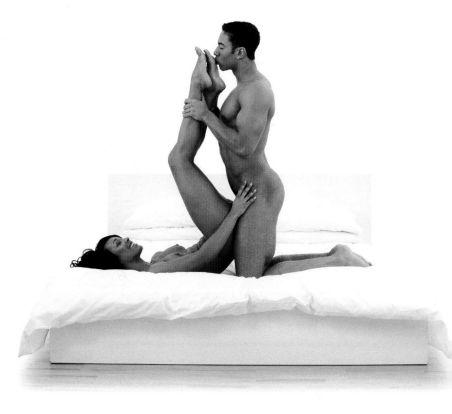

Kneel before her, and sprinkle her feet with kisses.

Perfect for: Awakening her to a spiritually uplifting experience.
Irresistible when: You continue your devotional all the way down her legs.

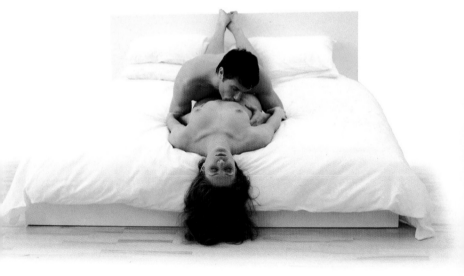

Seduce her with kisses while her head hangs over the edge of the bed.

Perfect for: Giving her a deliciously dizzying head rush.
Irresistible when: You nuzzle her beauty spot, and leave her on a cliffhanger.

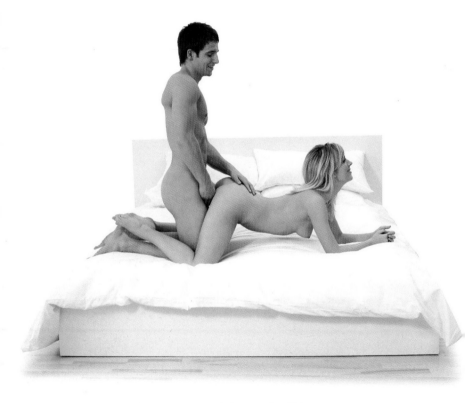

Cover your glans in lube, and twirl it on her anus.

Perfect for: Slippery sensations that open her up.
Irresistible when: You caress the small of her back with your palm.

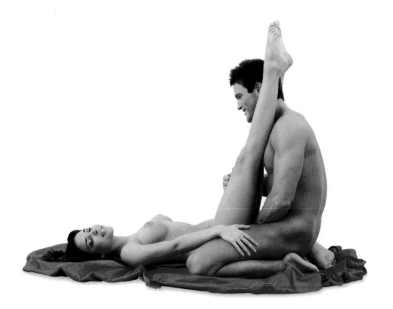

Take your drill bit in your hand, and swirl it on the opening of her well.

Perfect for: Making her hot and wet.
Irresistible when: You use your fingers to make her greedy for more.

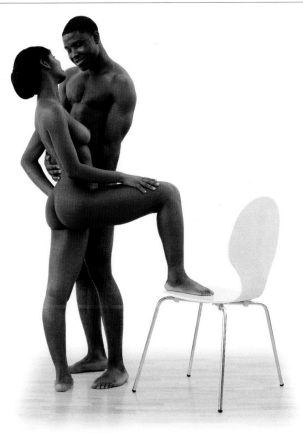

Greet her by sliding your fingers over her pubes and between her legs.

Perfect for: Giving her an X-rated how-do-you-do.
Irresistible when: Your fingers stay put, and you introduce her to your lips.

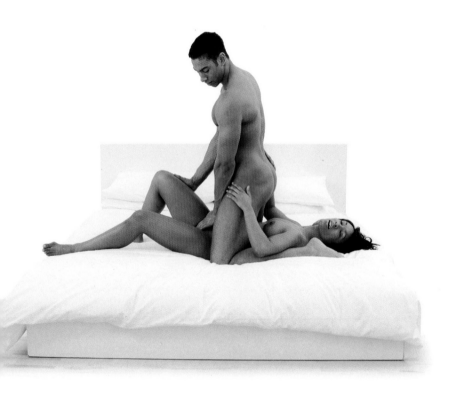

Kneel astride her, and caress her flower with your fingertips.

Perfect for: When she's in the mood to be plucked.
Irresistible when: You give her daisy kisses all around her garden.

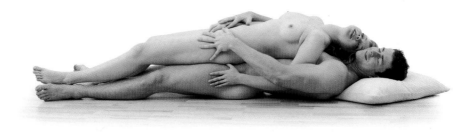

Lie her on top, then take her hand and slide it between her legs.

Perfect for: Making her feel lovingly embraced, but not crowded.
Irresistible when: You move your hand on hers in an intoxicating rhythm.

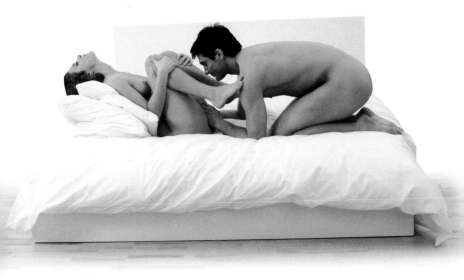

Ask her to pull her knees up to her chest for some hot sexploration.

Perfect for: Making her delirious with pleasure as you map her hot spots.
Irresistible when: You bend your fingers in a come-here gesture on her G-spot.

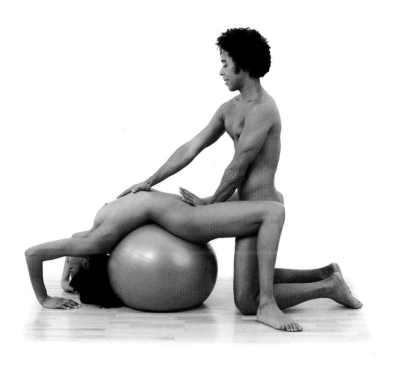

Apply firm hand pressure to her torso, and pelvis while she's upside-down.

Perfect for: Adding an erotic frisson to her yoga practice.
Irresistible when: Your thumb makes intimate friends with her G-spot.

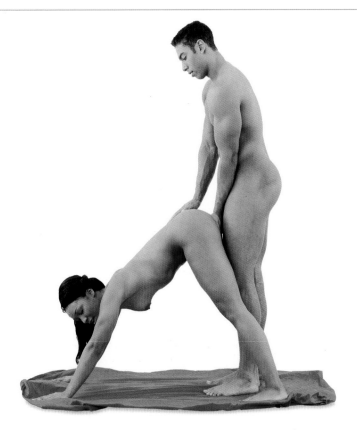

Arrange her in this classic pose, then get naughty with your hands.

Perfect for: Hot sensations to make her yelp.
Irresistible when: You throw yourself into some heavy petting.

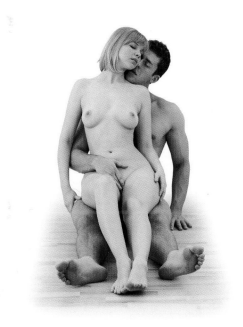

Sit her down, and offer her your finest handiwork.

Perfect for: When she wants to close her eyes, and fantasize.
Irresistible when: You talk dirty in her ear.

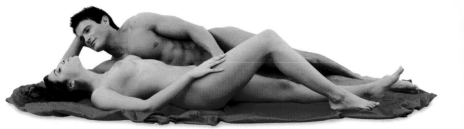

Slip your hand between her legs while you're cuddling in bed.

Perfect for: Playful canoodling that gathers momentum.
Irresistible when: She sets the pace, and you match it.

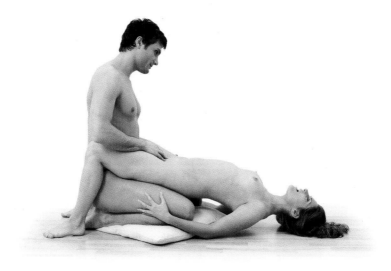

Let her lie back on your lap for easy, hand–to–clitoris access.

Perfect for: Sizzling sensations that give her spasms of desire.
Irresistible when: You slide your fingers slickly inside her.

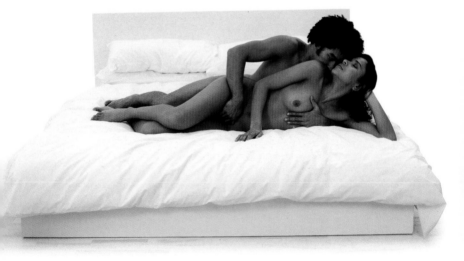

Twine your arms around her, so you're touching both bases.

Perfect for: Making her libido soar until she just can't contain it.
Irresistible when: You press your hot lips against her neck and ear lobe.

155 Nipping her nips

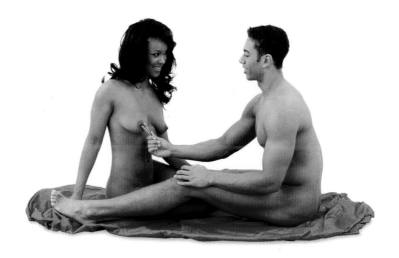

Deliver some home-made erotic torture—pinch her nipples with clothespins.

Perfect for: When she demands spontaneous sadism.
Irresistible when: You keep your clamping experiment short and sweet.

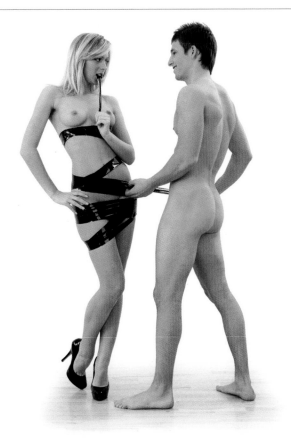

Twine bondage tape around her body while she holds the end between her teeth.

Perfect for: When strapping her up makes her sap rise.
Irresistible when: You caress her longingly through the gaps.

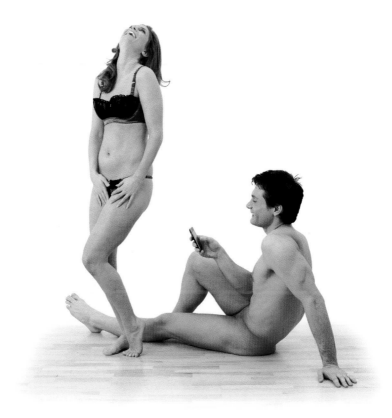

Trigger a remote-controlled vibrator in her panties by calling her from your phone.

Perfect for: Making her feel lip-bitingly aroused.
Irresistible when: You use it to seduce her when you're out of town.

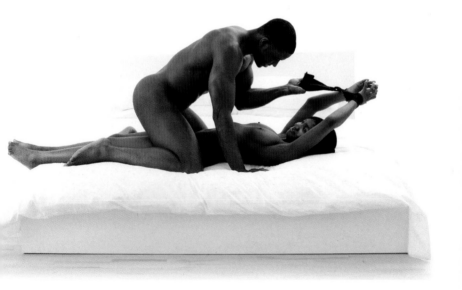

Gently wind a silk scarf around her wrists, then raise her arms over her head.

Perfect for: Making her a receiver rather than a giver.
Irresistible when: Your caresses make her arch and writhe in ecstasy.

151 Tush teasing

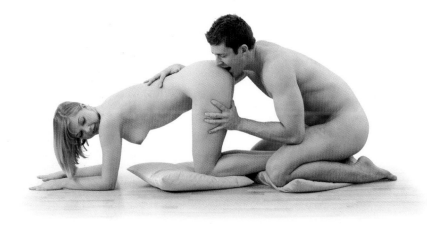

Breathe hotly on her bottom.

Perfect for: Giving her cheeks a warm, sexy glow.
Irresistible when: You stay put, and steam up other local hot spots.

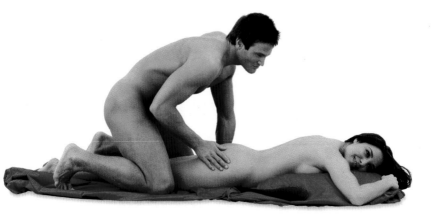

Turn gentle after you've spanked her. Soothe her stinging cheeks with a massage.

Perfect for: Making her say, "Mmmmm".
Irresistible when: You reach for the paddle again with a wicked glint in your eye.

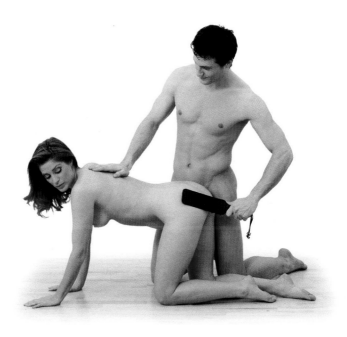

Pat her firmly on her cheek with a specially-made paddle.

Perfect for: When surrendering control makes her moist.
Irresistible when: The vibrations travel to her front bottom.

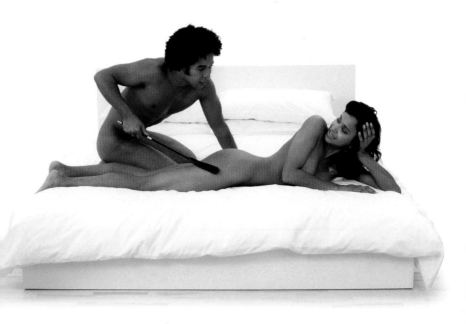

Stroke her thighs and buttocks with a riding crop.

Perfect for: Giving her that kinky feeling of being kept in check.
Irresistible when: You add some brisk spanks to your horseplay.

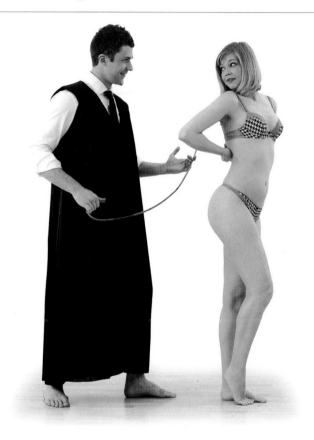

Be her lusty cane-wielding headmaster.

Perfect for: Giving her some X-rated private tutoring.
Irresistible when: You reward good behavior with sexual favors.

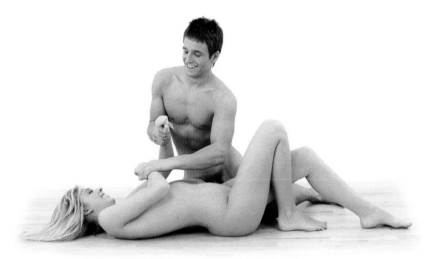

Hold her wrists, and playfully challenge her to escape.

Perfect for: Suddenly making her pulse race.
Irresistible when: Your tussle ends up in a passionate, breathless romp.

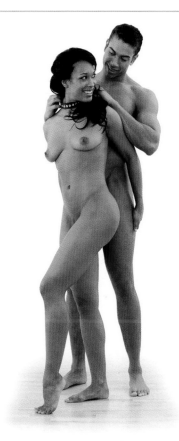

Circle her neck with a studded collar, and prepare to dominate her.

Perfect for: Stroking her all over, just the way she likes it.
Irresistible when: You attach a leash to her collar, and take her for a walk.

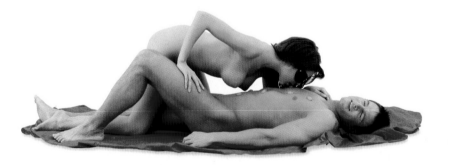

Blindfold her, and ask her to find the grapes, dabs of honey, and chocolate chips.

Perfect for: The delight of discovering new territories.
Irresistible when: You swap roles, and thoroughly explore her juicy bits too.

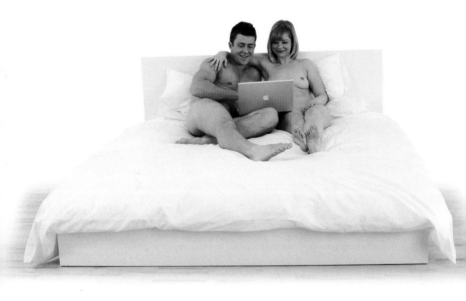

Give her a choice of X-rated movies to watch.

Perfect for: Making her feel deliciously rude and daring.
Irresistible when: You can't keep your hands off her during the movie.

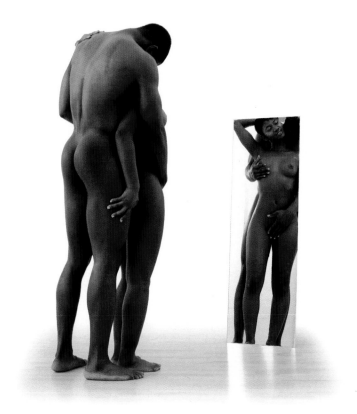

Stimulate her in front of a mirror, so she can enjoy the reflected glory.

Perfect for: Letting her see how gorgeous she looks.
Irresistible when: You make her so excited that you fall to the floor together.

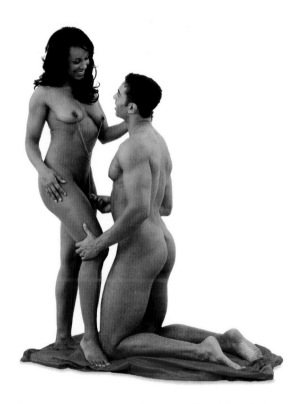

Pop some clamps on her, then gently tweak her chain.

Perfect for: Making her say "Ow", but in a good way.
Irresistible when: You take her to the peak of the pain/pleasure threshold.

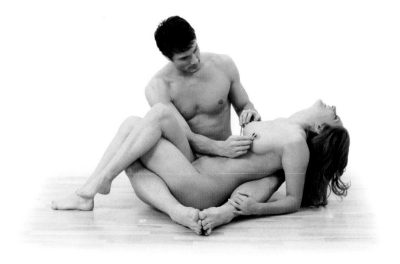

Gently apply clamps to her nipples.

Perfect for: When professional pinching drenches her with desire.
Irresistible when: You perk up her nipples with an ice cube beforehand.

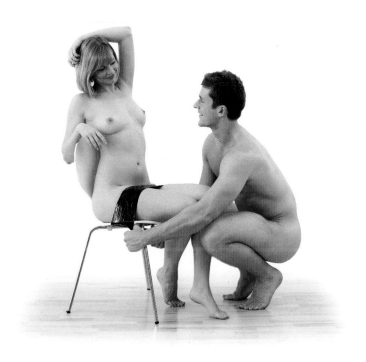

Use bondage tape to keep her chair-bound.

Perfect for: Lavishing her body with sexual treats she can't refuse.
Irresistible when: You take her to the peak of arousal before setting her free.

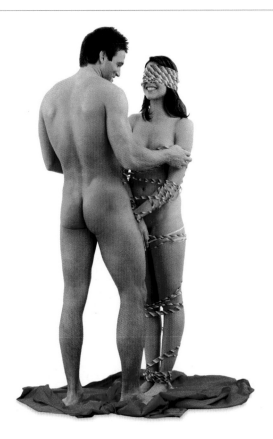

Tie her up with something she can easily get out of—ribbons or paper streamers.

Perfect for: Piquing her interest, and preparing her for Kink Level 2.
Irresistible when: You buy her fluffy handcuffs as a graduation present.

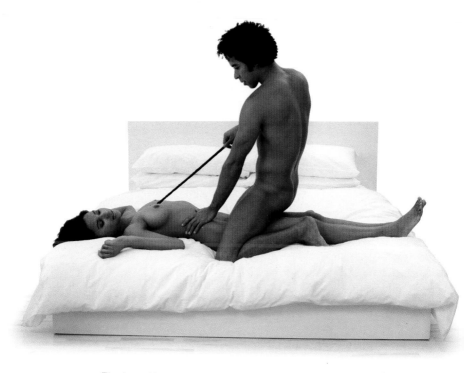

Play her strict teacher. Tease her with the tip of your cane.

Perfect for: When she likes to feel the weight of your authority.
Irresistible when: You introduce the tip of your other stick too.

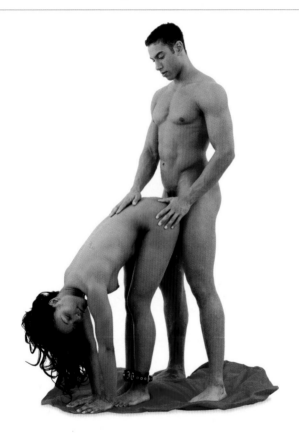

Play master and slave—bind her ankles, and bend her over.

Perfect for: When she's in the mood for some sexy violation.
Irresistible when: You whip her with your slave-driver.

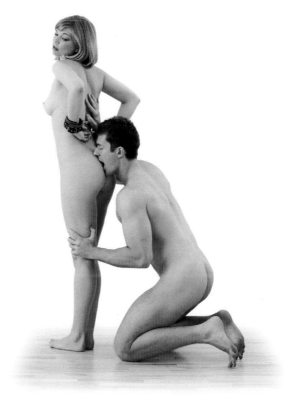

Handcuff her, then bite and nibble her buttocks.

Perfect for: Pleasure she can't escape from.
Irresistible when: You slip your tongue between her cheeks.

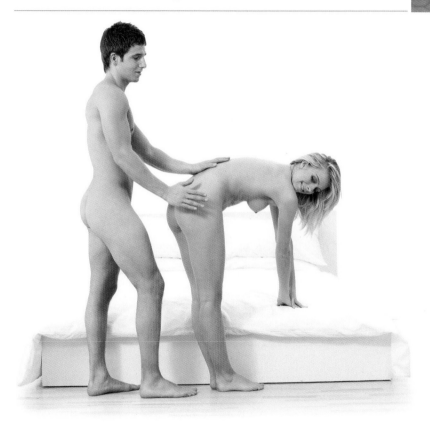

Fix her with a steely look, and tell her to bend over.

Perfect for: When submission makes her head spin.
Irresistible when: Your palm makes a powerful and pleasing landing.

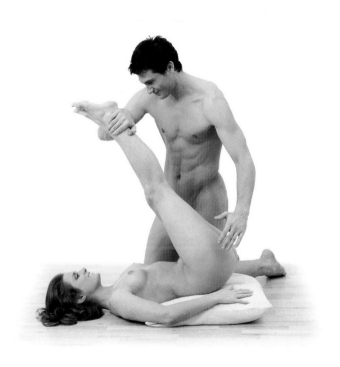

Lift her legs, and spank her in the "you've-been-a-naughty-girl" position.

Perfect for: Experimenting with dominance and submission.
Irresistible when: You mix it up with some caring clitoral caresses.

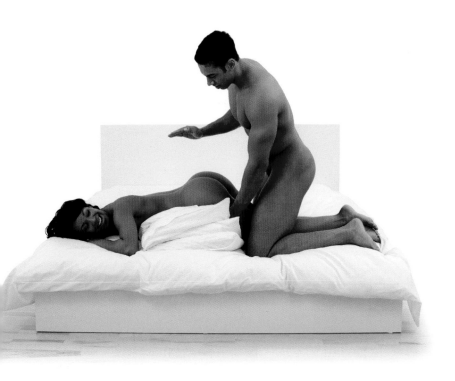

Lay her on a ramp of cushions for an extended spanking session.

Perfect for: Exposed vulnerability that makes her gasp.
Irresistible when: You target the spasm-spot where her thighs meet her bottom.

131 Hot cross buns

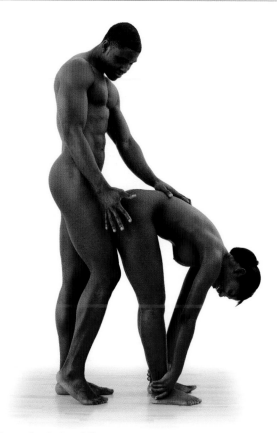

Challenge her to touch her toes, then surprise her with a spank.

Perfect for: Delivering a hot sting that makes her throb.
Irresistible when: You use your passion baton on her cheeks too.

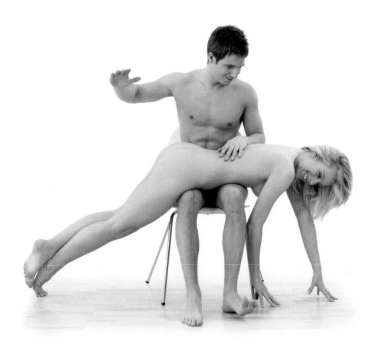

Put her over your knee, and give her your best spank.

Perfect for: When she needs some firm discipline.
Irresistible when: You keep going until she begs you to stop.

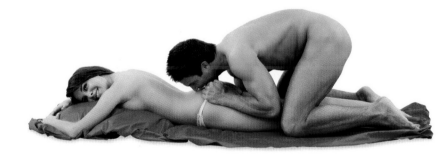

Give her a secret love bite.

Perfect for: A going-away gift she'll love to look back on.
Irresistible when: You give her a matching one on the other cheek.

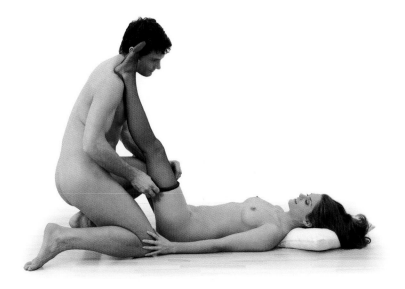

Slowly unroll her stocking while gazing into her eyes.

Perfect for: Conveying your naughty intentions.
Irresistible when: You plant feather-light kisses along the inside of her leg.

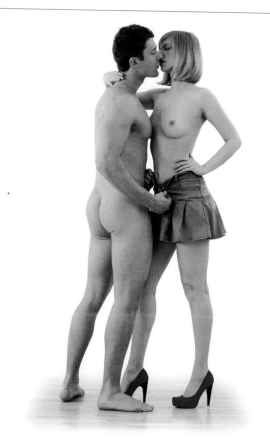

Undress her with practiced ease while kissing her.

Perfect for: Giving her a smoldering got-to-have-you-now vibe.
Irresistible when: You cup her bottom in your hands as her skirt falls to the floor.

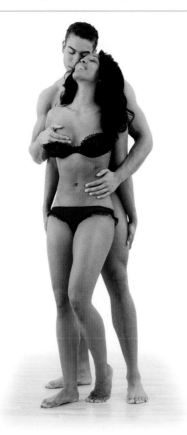

Slip your hand inside her bra to fondle her assets.

Perfect for: A sneaky nipple tweak to prompt her passion.
Irresistible when: You've got one hand in each cup.

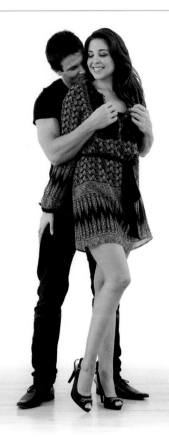

Nuzzle her neck while your fingers make light work of her buttons.

Perfect for: Pausing to play with her peaks on the way.
Irresistible when: You moan passionately as her dress slides down her body.

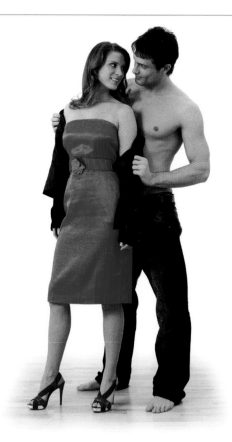

Do the chivalrous thing, and help her take her coat off.

Perfect for: Enticing her with some old-school charm.
Irresistible when: You offer to slip her dress off, too.

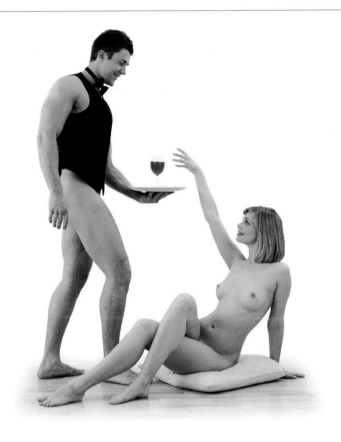

Be her kinky butler. Wait on her hand and foot.

Perfect for: Letting her give you orders, and ogle you at the same time.
Irresistible when: You say "Can I be of *personal* service, Madam?"

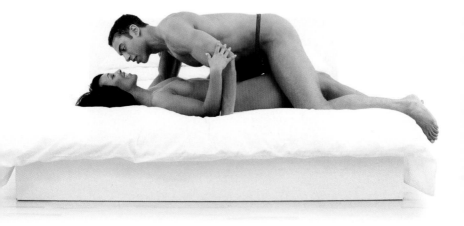

Squeeze your beast into an animal-print thong, and go on the prowl.

Perfect for: When she wants to be chased and ravaged.
Irresistible when: You bury your face between her legs to find her hidden dragon.

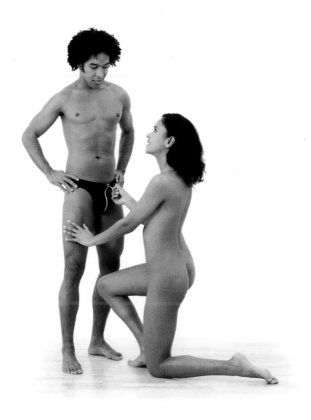

121 Zipper zeal

Strip down to a pert posing pouch, and invite her to unleash the boys.

Perfect for: When she loves the unwrapping part.
Irresistible when: You spring out to greet her.

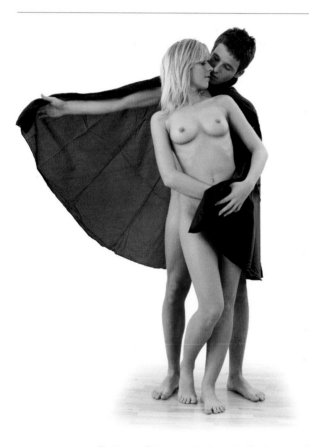

Swirl your Batman cloak seductively around her.

Perfect for: The thrill of being within your superpower.
Irresistible when: You say "Quick, put your hands on my Bat-rope".

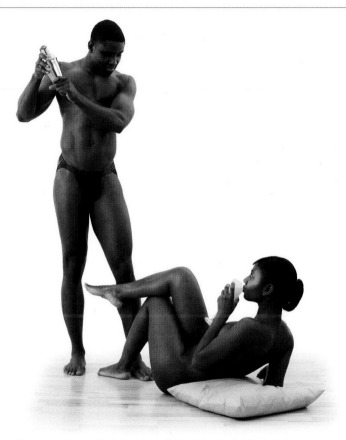

Be her sexy cocktail waiter—mix her favorite liquid refreshment.

Perfect for: Firing up her mood on a quiet Friday evening.
Irresistible when: You invite her to start the weekend with a bang.

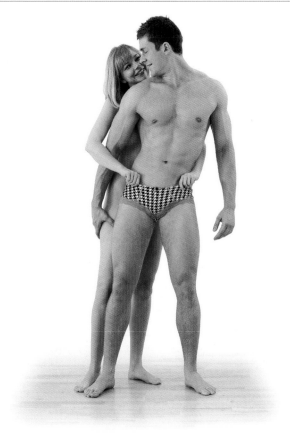

Ask her to dress you in a pair of her panties.

Perfect for: Letting her enjoy the glorious, phallus-hugging display.
Irresistible when: Your stallion breaks out of its constraints.

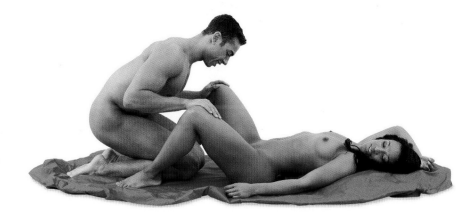

117 Peep beau

Pause for a second to moan your appreciation before going down on her.

Perfect for: Giving her a gorgeously lickable feeling.
Irresistible when: You sigh with sensual satisfaction on arrival.

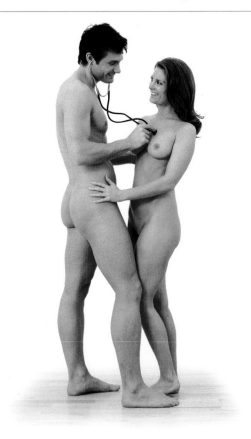

As her doctor, measure how fast her heart is beating.

Perfect for: Discovering how excited she is by your stethoscope.
Irresistible when: You do something unexpected to make her pulse race.

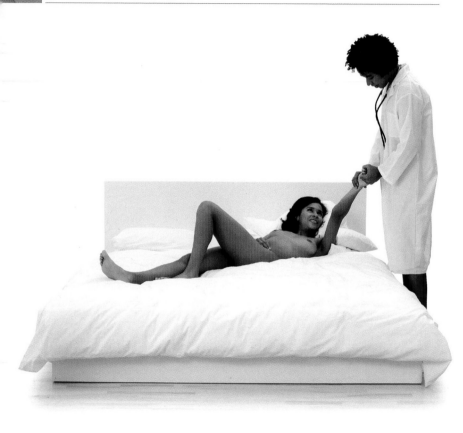

Slip on a white coat, and give her a top-to-toe check-up.

Perfect for: When she's writhing and feverish.
Irresistible when: You soothe her inflamed parts with your healing hands.

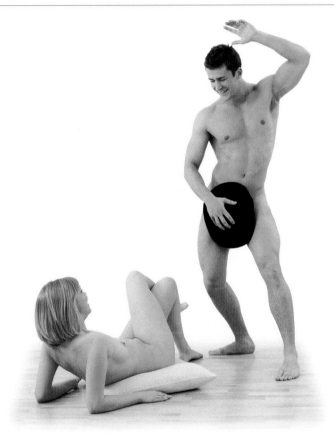

Dance naked for her, but leave one gorgeous thing to her imagination.

Perfect for: Letting her fantasize as you do your sexiest moves.
Irresistible when: You playfully throw your hat in the air.

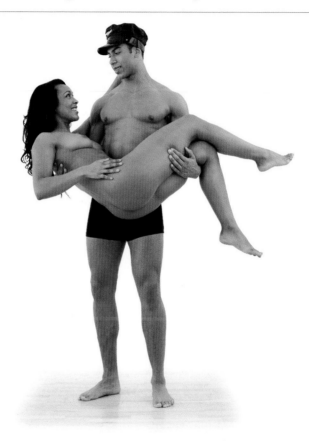

Pick her up *Officer and a Gentleman*-style, and carry her to bed.

Perfect for: Thrilling her with want-you-right-now urgency.
Irresistible when: You kiss, and carry her at the same time.

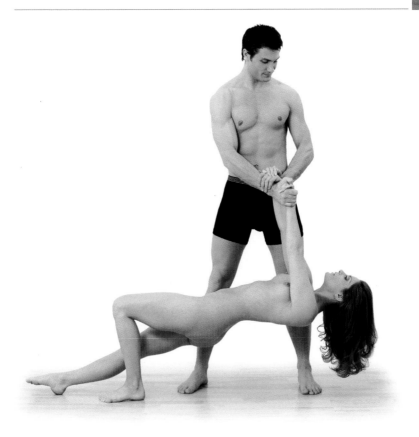

Make her heart race with a floor-brushing salsa drop.

Perfect for: Giving her an intense whole-body rush.
Irresistible when: You gaze down at her with smoldering Latin lust.

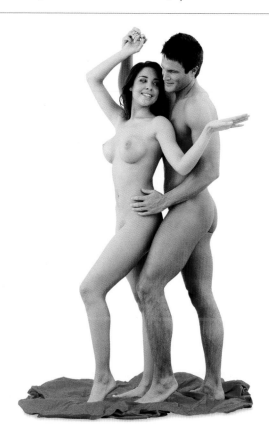

Slide your hand around her waist, and spin her to some hot mambo.

Perfect for: Building up a rhythmic intensity that leaves her breathless.
Irresistible when: You mesmerize her with your sexy Cuban hips.

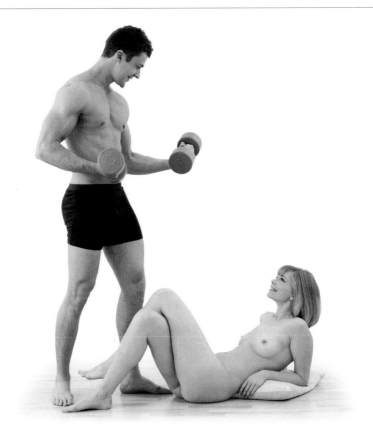

Work up a manly sweat before pouncing on her.

Perfect for: Making her want to suddenly lie down.
Irresistible when: You press your taut, hot, glossy skin against hers.

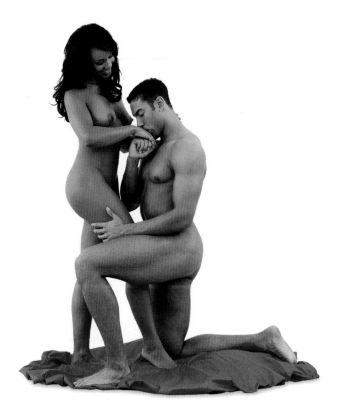

In true gentlemanly fashion, get down on one knee, and kiss her hand.

Perfect for: Charming the pants off her when you haven't seen her all day.
Irresistible when: You propose on sight.

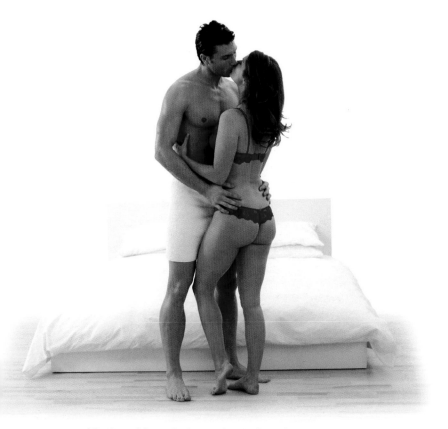

Kiss her while you're hot and moist from the shower.

Perfect for: Stirring early-morning ripples of passion.
Irresistible when: You pass her the phone, and tell her to call in late for work.

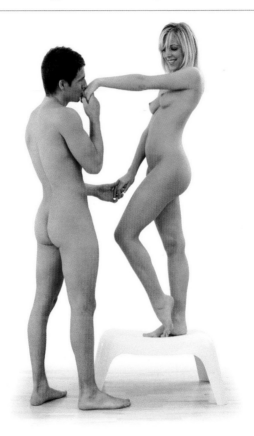

Help her up onto a stool, chair, or custom-made pedestal.

Perfect for: When you want to treat her like a lady.
Irresistible when: You carry her off to a satin-sheeted, four-poster bed.

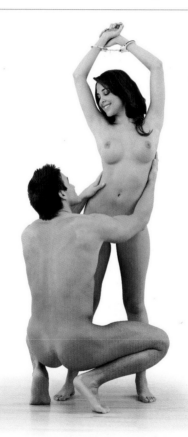

As an officer of the law it's your job to frisk her thoroughly.

Perfect for: When she's carrying inflammatory goods on her person.
Irresistible when: She feels the weight of your nightstick.

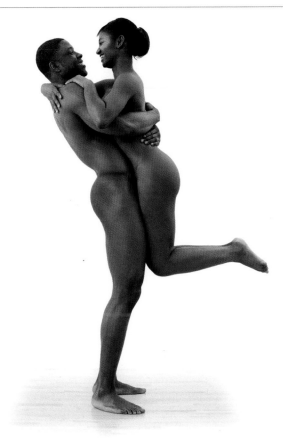

Take her breath away by spinning her around.

Perfect for: When you've got something to celebrate.
Irresistible when: You give her a mouth-merging, mid-spin kiss.

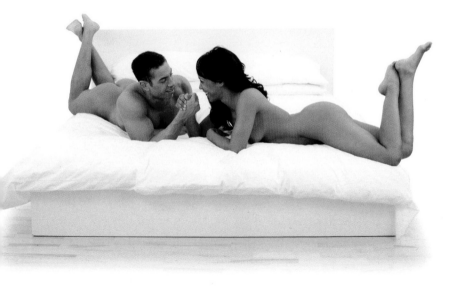

Grab her hand, and challenge her to an arm wrestle.

Perfect for: Arousing the feisty fighter in her.
Irresistible when: You let her win, and up the game to a full-body wrestle.

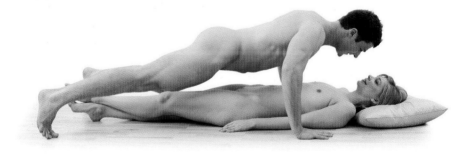

Work out on top of her. Try 50 muscle-popping push-ups.

Perfect for: Pumping movements that stir her loins, and fire her imagination.
Irresistible when: You "penetrate" her thighs with each thrust.

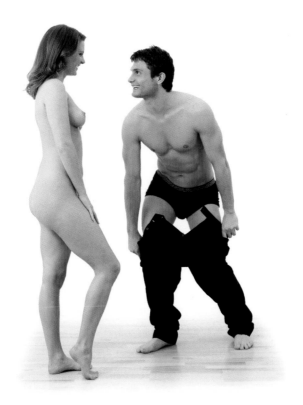

Slide your pants slowly down your thighs.

Perfect for: Giving her that got-to-get-my-hands-on-you feeling.
Irresistible when: You gyrate your hips to a hot, stripping anthem.

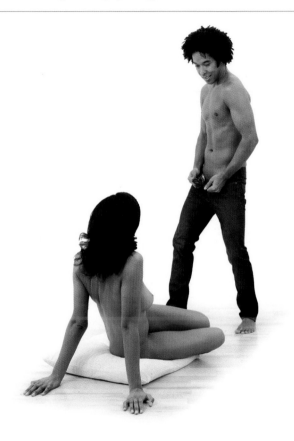

Be her sexy strippergram—slowly unbutton your fly.

Perfect for: When watching is her ultimate turn-on.
Irresistible when: In no rush at all, you ease your jeans over your hips…

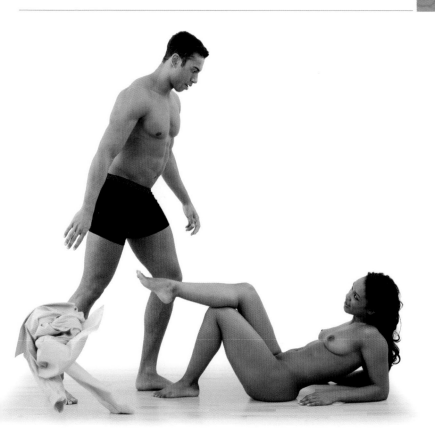

Rip your shirt off, and make your move.

Perfect for: When you know she's passion-starved.
Irresistible when: You pounce on her, then roll her over so she's on top.

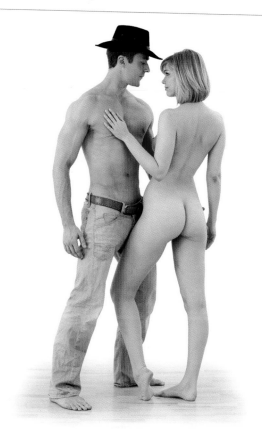

Treat her to your best cowboy impersonation.

Perfect for: When swaggering confidence makes her swoon.
Irresistible when: You ask her to undo your belt and zipper.

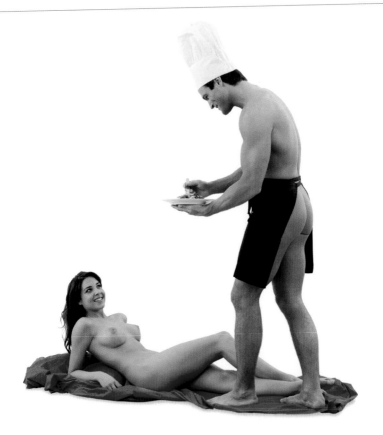

Slip into an apron and chef's hat, and seduce her with your fine cuisine.

Perfect for: Feeding her one, mouth-watering bite at a time.
Irresistible when: She spots the sausage under your apron.

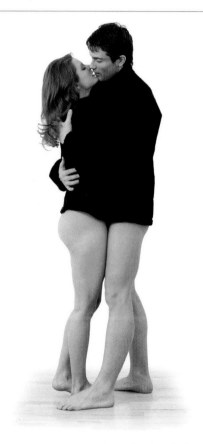

Hug and kiss her inside your baggy coat.

Perfect for: Sweet romance when she's feeling shivery.
Irresistible when: You pick her up, and kiss her passionately.

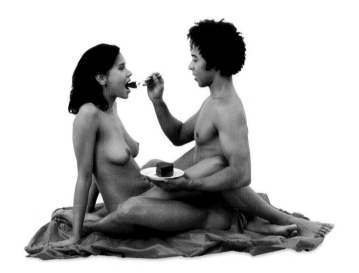

Feed her forkfuls of the finest chocolate cake.

Perfect for: Her birthday breakfast.
Irresistible when: You tenderly kiss the crumbs from her mouth.

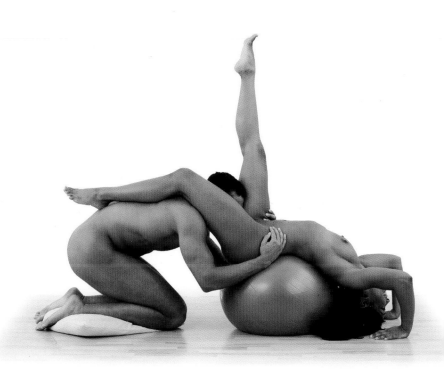

Curve your tongue around her while she's in a backbend.

Perfect for: Eye-popping sensations that arc through her body.
Irresistible when: Your ball game is fast and furious.

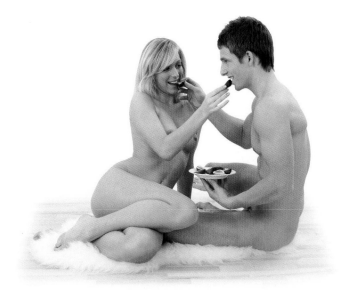

Press juicy figs into each other's mouths.

Perfect for: When she likes her summer picnics to turn naughty.
Irresistible when: You lean over, and lick fig juice from her lips.

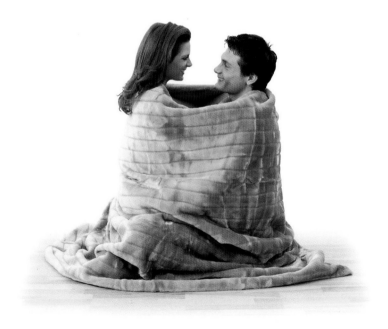

Cuddle her naked body underneath a huge, soft blanket.

Perfect for: Discreet gropes on the beach.
Irresistible when: You pull her undercover for a sensual snog.

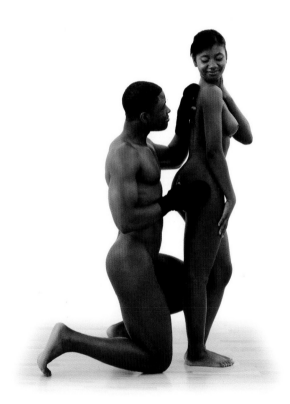

Caress her curves with some furry mittens.

Perfect for: Making her feel as soft and strokable as a pussycat.
Irresistible when: You play the tiger to her kitten.

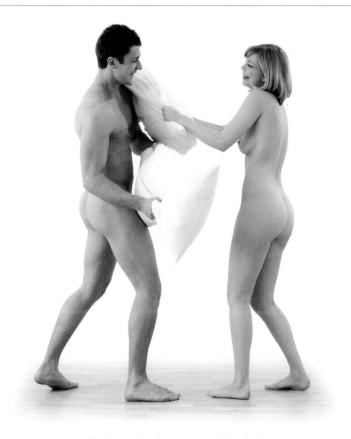

Challenge her to a wanton pillow fight.

Perfect for: An erotic way to work off her sexual tension.
Irresistible when: Action ends with you dropping the pillows for a naked romp.

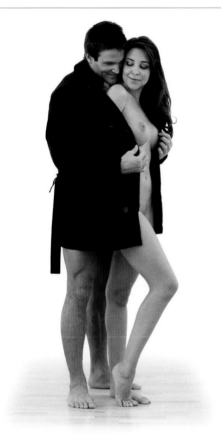

Be chivalrous: ask her to share your coat.

Perfect for: Making her feel sexily button-holed at the end of the night.
Irresistible when: You keep her tightly wrapped up all the way home.

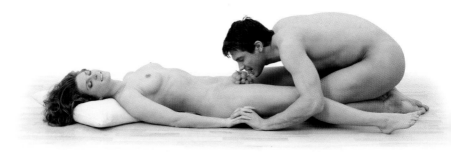

Eat grapes one by one from her Cupid's triangle.

Perfect for: Making her feel ripe for the picking.
Irresistible when: You bite into a grape, and let the juice trickle between her legs.

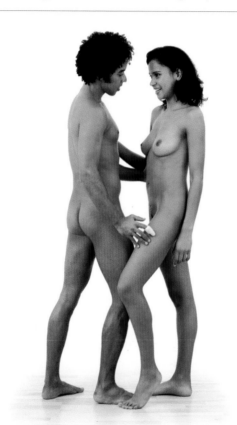

Wear a fingertip vibrator, and take your hand for a walk up her thigh.

Perfect for: Women who prefer small, sweet sex toys to huge, phallic ones.
Irresistible when: You reach destination clitoris.

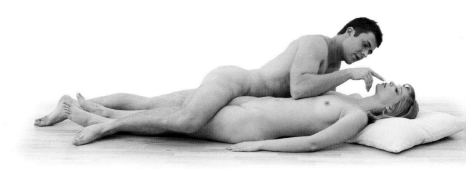

Drip honey, cream, or syrup onto her lips.

Perfect for: Heightening her senses of touch, and taste.
Irresistible when: You tenderly kiss the sweetness from her lips.

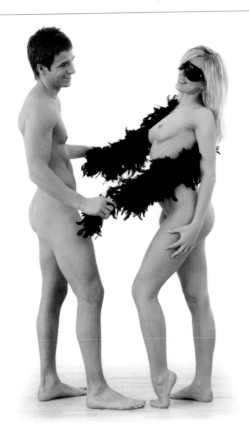

Blindfold her, then caress her body all over with a feather boa.

Perfect for: Enveloping her in soft and sensual luxury.
Irresistible when: You pull her toward you, and feather her moan-making spots.

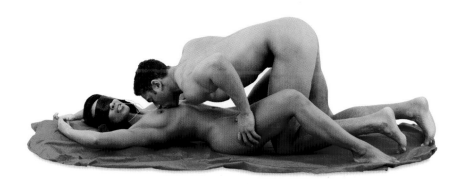

Deprive her of sight, wire her up to some slinky tunes, and set about servicing her.

Perfect for: Letting her enter the blissful realm of her senses.
Irresistible when: You give her a firm "No" if she tries to reciprocate.

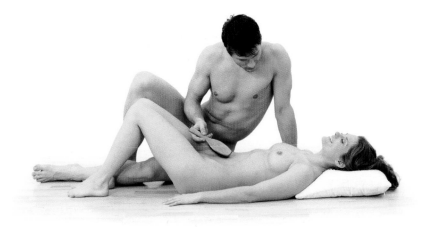

Give her a novel type of touch—tickle her skin with a hairbrush.

Perfect for: Making her bristle with arousal.
Irresistible when: You slide the brush down, and offer to groom her curls.

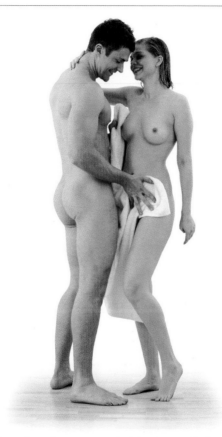

Catch her when she comes out of the shower. Be her personal dryer.

Perfect for: A sensual beginning to a night of lust.
Irresistible when: You insist on lingering over her wettest bits.

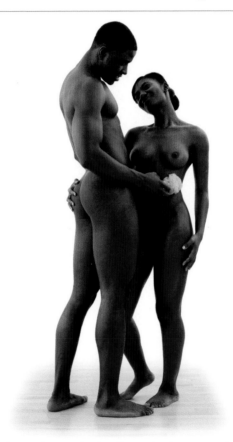

Caress her wet body with a natural sponge or loofah.

Perfect for: Giving her sexy shudders in the shower.
Irresistible when: You squeeze warm water onto her Bermuda Triangle.

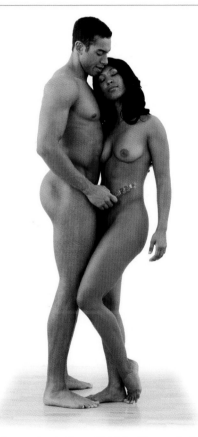

Roll a glass dildo over her belly, and let it find its way between her legs.

Perfect for: Exquisite sensations exactly where she wants them.
Irresistible when: You've warmed the glass first.

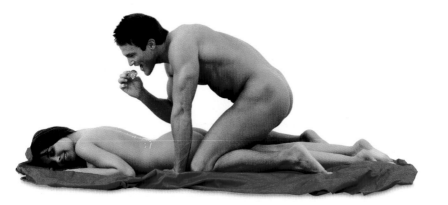

Drizzle her with cream, then twirl your strawberries on her.

Perfect for: Adult-only picnics in the bedroom.
Irresistible when: You pounce on her, and make strawberry smoothie.

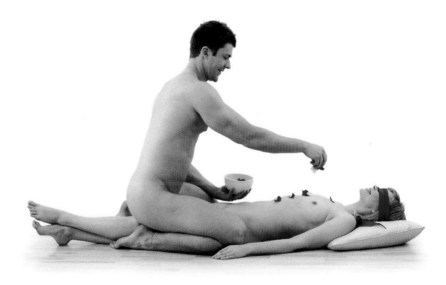

Cover her eyes with a silk scarf, and scatter rose petals on her skin.

Perfect for: Velvet rain sensations.
Irresistible when: You fill the room with flickering candlelight.

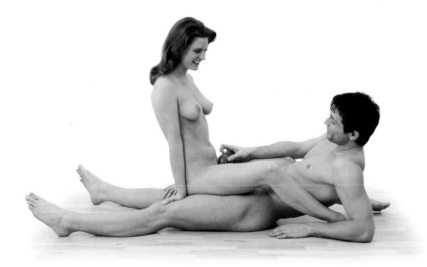

Press a pebble vibrator between her legs.

Perfect for: When round, curvy sex toys press her buttons perfectly.
Irresistible when: You move it at just the speed and rhythm she likes.

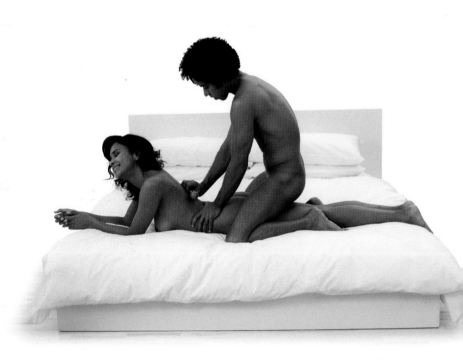

Relax her with a plug-in, tension-relieving massager—a.k.a. the prude's vibrator.

Perfect for: Turning her to putty in your hands.
Irresistible when: You let the vibrator stray into her erotic quarter.

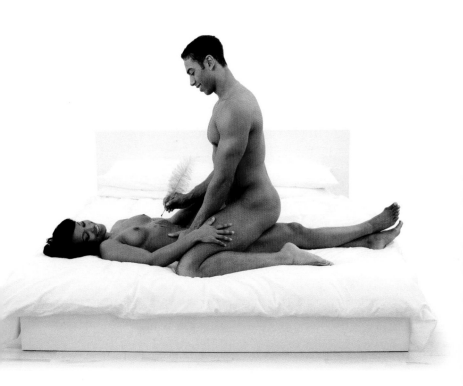

Use a quill to decorate her body with chocolate-flavored body paint.

Perfect for: Making her back arch with skin-teasing tickles.
Irresistible when: You lay down your quill, and feast upon her body.

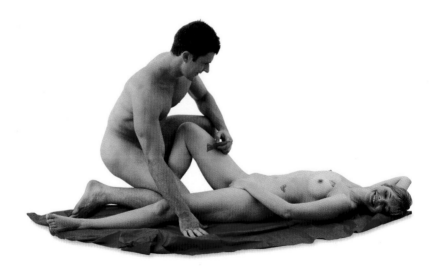

Use a body pen to mark out her erogenous zones.

Perfect for: Making her realize how much you adore her body.
Irresistible when: You write a saucy message on her naughty bits.

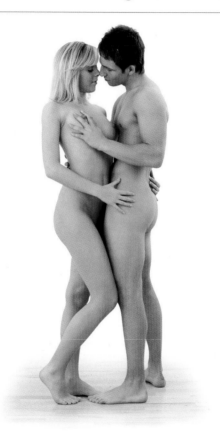

Press her nipple between your index and middle finger.

Perfect for: Sending erotic currents up and down her body.
Irresistible when: You let your fingers tweak, and your tongue flick.

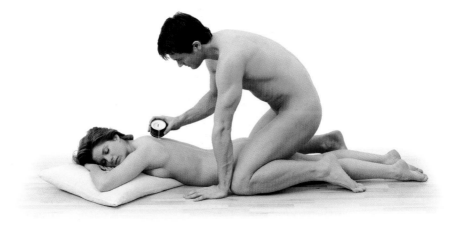

Snuff out the flame of a massage candle, and drip the warm wax onto her skin.

Perfect for: Giving her a hot, tactile treat.
Irresistible when: You rub in the wax with slow, seductive strokes.

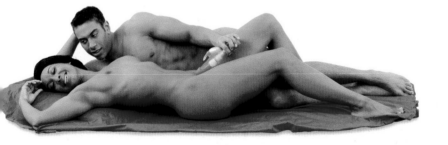

Caress her with the legendary, battery-powered rabbit.

Perfect for: A magic touch that leaves her spellbound.
Irresistible when: You give her an abracadabra moment by switching it to max.

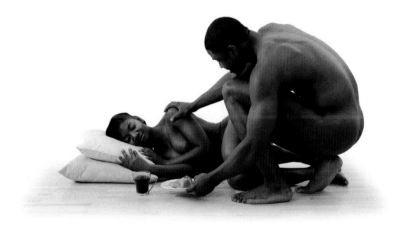

Wake her up with freshly brewed coffee and her favorite breakfast.

Perfect for: Filling her with warm, sleepy gratitude.
Irresistible when: You climb back into bed, and wake her up properly.

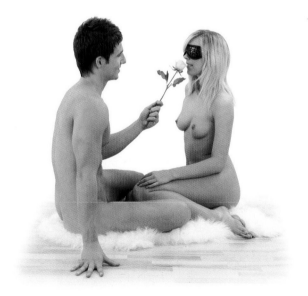

Blindfold her, then waft a scented rose under her nose.

Perfect for: A fragrant, flowery seduction.
Irresistible when: You sing a romantic ballad at the same time.

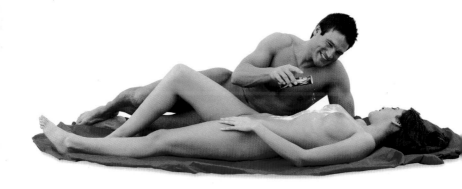

Sprinkle edible body dust on her joy spots.

Perfect for: Subtle sensations that make her feel yummy.
Irresistible when: You give her a long and thorough licking.

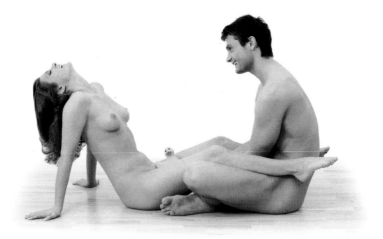

Tease her love triangle with a vibrating rubber duck.

Perfect for: Getting out of the bathtub with a smile.
Irresistible when: You make her giggle her way to a climax.

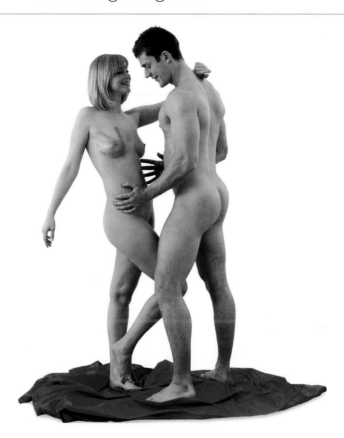

Manhandle her with gold body paint.

Perfect for: When she loves the sight of your hands all over her body.
Irresistible when: You pull her lustfully to the floor, and smudge your paintwork.

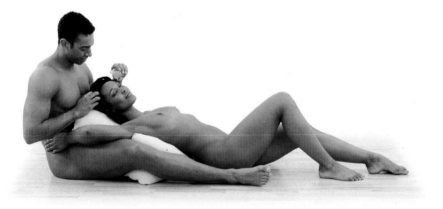

Drizzle coconut oil onto her scalp, and rake it through her hair with your fingertips.

Perfect for: Planting hot, tropical fantasies in her head.
Irresistible when: You play the part of her adoring island lover.

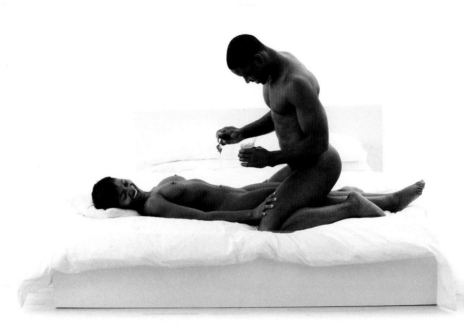

Lay her down, and drip honey into her navel.

Perfect for: Making her feel deliciously moist and sticky.
Irresistible when: You lap it all up with a soft tongue.

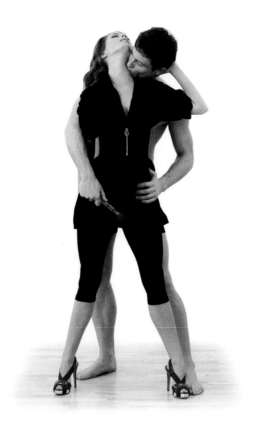

Press a vibrator between her legs.

Perfect for: Putting a spring in her step before she goes out.
Irresistible when: You turn the vibe dial up to maximum.

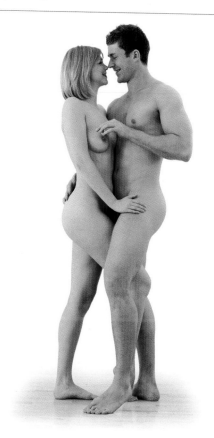

Rub oil into her breast, then circle an ice cube around her nipple.

Perfect for: The tantalizing sensation of oil and water trickling south.
Irresistible when: You warm up her nipple by sucking it.

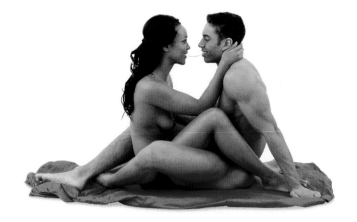

Share a strand of spaghetti. Suck until you meet in the middle.

Perfect for: A saucy ending to a romantic Italian dinner.
Irresistible when: You skip the cannoli and kiss instead.

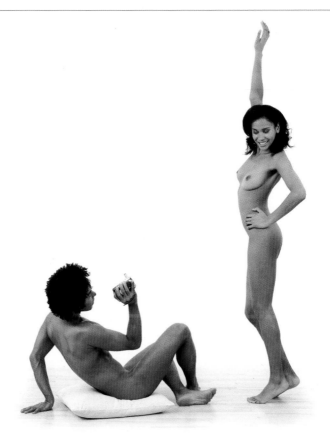

She's so hot that you have to record her.

Perfect for: Bringing out her sexy, exhibitionist side.
Irresistible when: You shoot ONLY her most flattering angles.

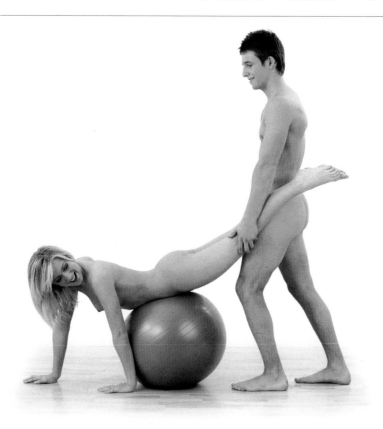

Sneak up, and take advantage of her during her Pilates practice.

Perfect for: Making a slinky appearance between her thighs.
Irresistible when: You ask to inspect her core muscles.

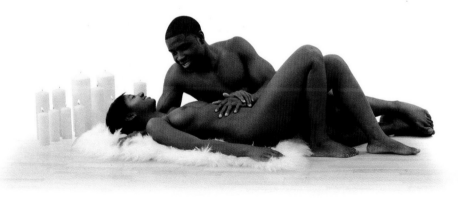

Make an erotic den for her with a fur rug, candles, and music.

Perfect for: A romantic reunion to make her swoon.
Irresistible when: You say "Your wish is my command".

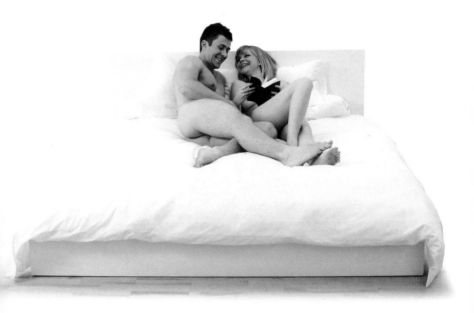

Take the *Kama Sutra* to bed with you.

Perfect for: Getting her in the mood for some red-hot positions.
Irresistible when: You ask her to pick something she's never done before.

A floral temptation

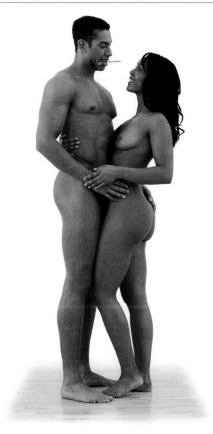

Risk a mouth full of thorns to give her the gift of a rose.

Perfect for: Romantic, post-fight make-ups.
Irresistible when: You sweep her off her feet in a passionate tango.

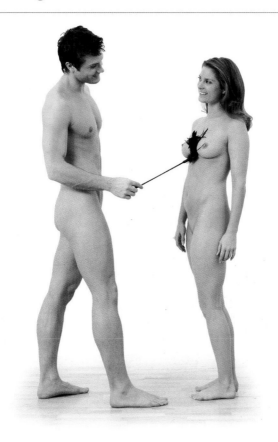

Tickle her breasts with a feather duster.

Perfect for: Titillation that makes her giggle.
Irresistible when: You ask which part of her body you should polish next.

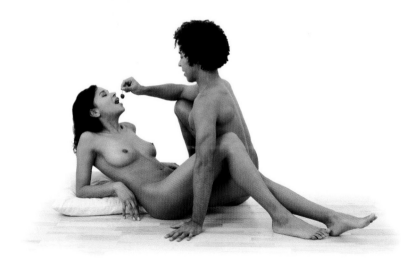

Dangle your ripest cherry in front of her lips.

Perfect for: Tempting her with something plump and juicy.
Irresistible when: She takes it in her mouth, and passes it back to you with a kiss.

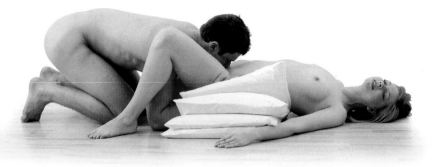

Slide some soft pillows under her before you go down on her.

Perfect for: Opening her up to oral pleasure.
Irresistible when: You passionately French kiss her bliss button.

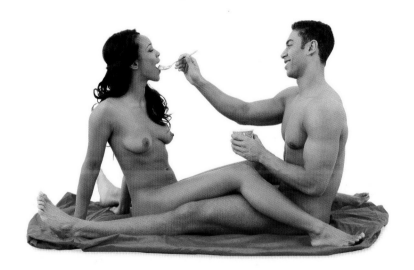

Teasingly feed her ice cream from a spoon.

Perfect for: Chilled-out flirting that makes her melt inside.
Irresistible when: Oops, you miss her mouth, and have to lick her clean.

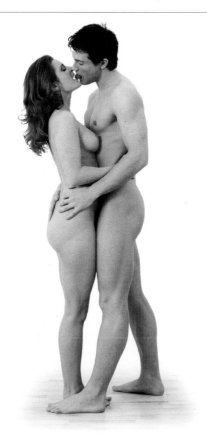

Deliver a strawberry by mouth as you kiss her.

Perfect for: Summer fruit picking.
Irresistible when: You get raunchy on a haystack afterward.

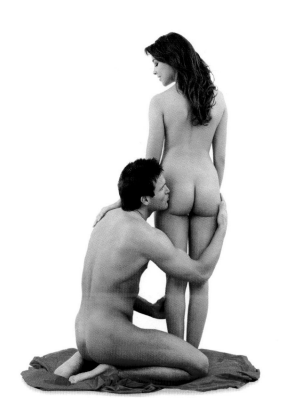

Lavish hot kisses on her muscle cakes.

Perfect for: An amorous feast when you pull down her panties.
Irresistible when: You circle your palm on her buns, too.

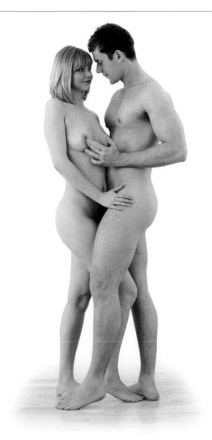

Oil your fingers, then move them in seductive spirals on her breasts.

Perfect for: Sending erotic currents downstairs.
Irresistible when: You devote special attention to her nipples.

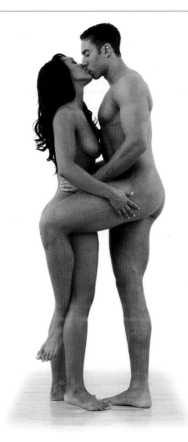

Clasp her tightly, wrap your leg around hers, and lock lips.

Perfect for: A naughty "you're-not-going-anywhere" vibe.
Irresistible when: You pull her to the floor, and do it horizontally.

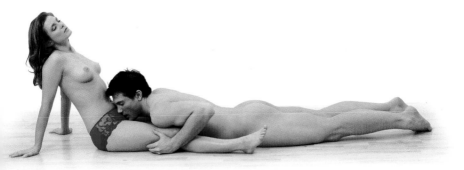

Get her steamed up by breathing hotly through her panties.

Perfect for: Setting her ablaze when it's cold outside.
Irresistible when: You take the direct approach, and warm her with your tongue.

47 Letting things slide

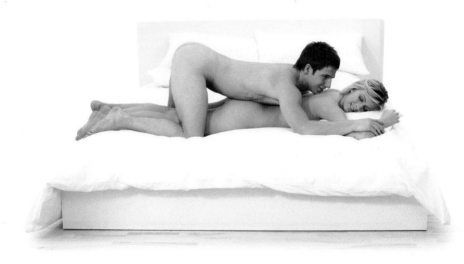

Oil your pecs, then slither your way up her bottom and back.

Perfect for: Giving her a sweet and slippery embrace.
Irresistible when: You come to rest with your snake firmly between her thighs.

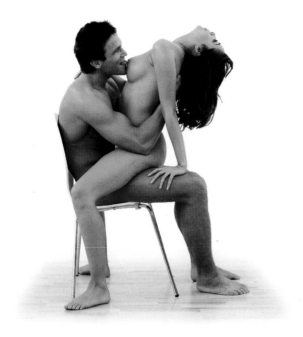

Drive her wild with the tip of your tongue on her nipples.

Perfect for: Making her desire blossom early.
Irresistible when: You whisper that you can't get enough of her.

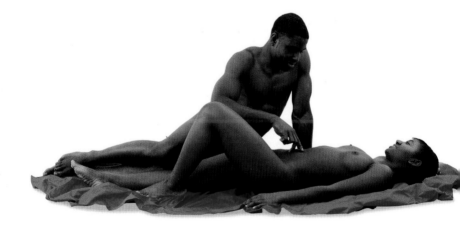

Take your fingers for a tantalizing walk over her navel, and belly.

Perfect for: Giving her butterflies in her tummy.
Irresistible when: Your fingers flutter down to her treasure box.

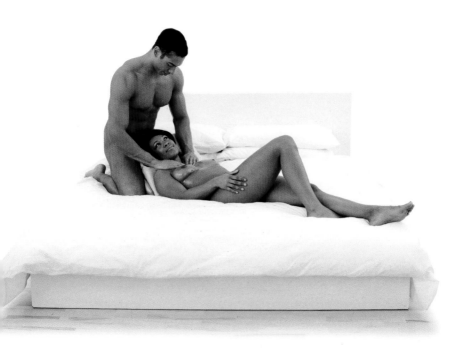

Make her chest slick with oil, then take your palms for a swim on her breasts.

Perfect for: Drenching her in desire.
Irresistible when: You dive smoothly down the middle of her body.

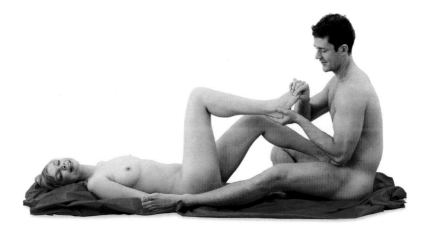

Oil your fingers, and slide them smoothly between her toes. Squeeze gently.

Perfect for: Making her say "Mmmmmm" at the end of a long day.
Irresistible when: Your massaging hand finds its way up her calf and thigh.

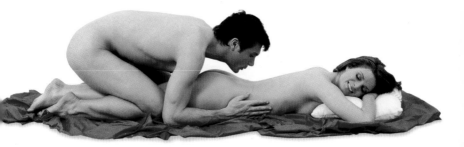

Blow a stream of warm air down the length of her spine.

Perfect for: Giving her shivers of pure delight.
Irresistible when: You slowly lick along the length of her spine, then blow her dry.

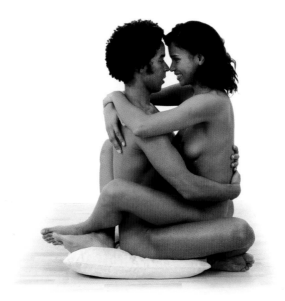

Sit her on your lap, wrap your arms around her, and nudge noses.

Perfect for: Making her feel like the most desirable woman on Earth.
Irresistible when: You grab her bottom, and pull her tightly onto your hardware.

Bunny strokes 40

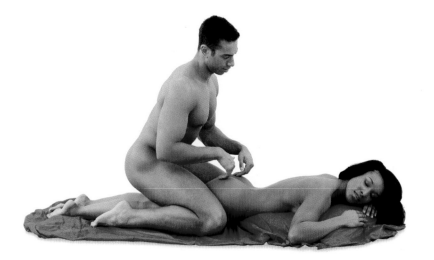

Lightly drag your claws over her mounds.

Perfect for: Making her tail twitch with pleasure.
Irresistible when: You introduce a rampant rabbit to shake things up.

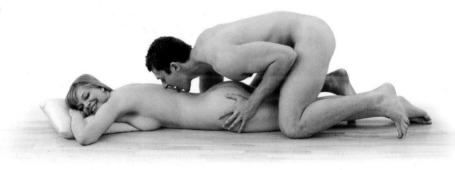

Slide up her body, sprinkling her skin with sensual licks and slow kisses.

Perfect for: Taking her to quivering heights of pleasure.
Irresistible when: You reach her ear and whisper "Turn over".

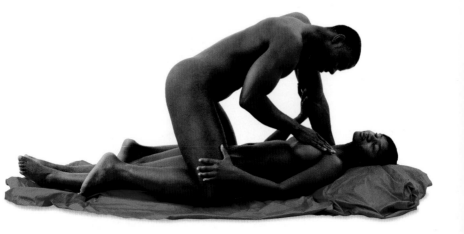

Smooth your oiled palm up and over the whole of her breast.

Perfect for: Blissful, taken-in-hand sensations.
Irresistible when: You catch her nipple between your fingers as you go.

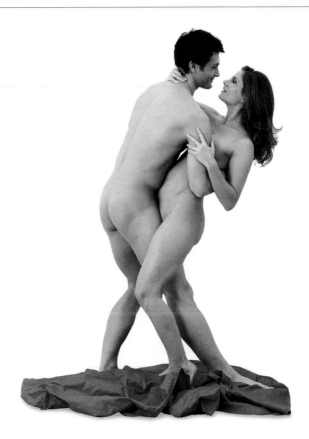

Let her bump against the hardness of your thigh.

Perfect for: Sexy seductions on the dance floor.
Irresistible when: You move in time to lust-making music.

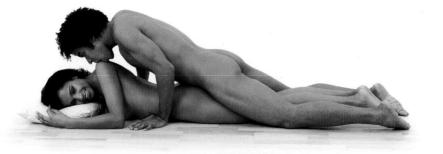

Pounce on her, and tiger-bite her shoulders and back.

Perfect for: Wowing her with your wild side.
Irresistible when: You flip her over, and give into your animal urges.

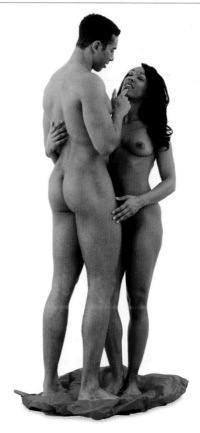

Ask her to close her eyes, and softly trace the shape of her lips with your finger.

Perfect for: The heart-fluttering moments before a kiss.
Irresistible when: You moisten your finger on her tongue.

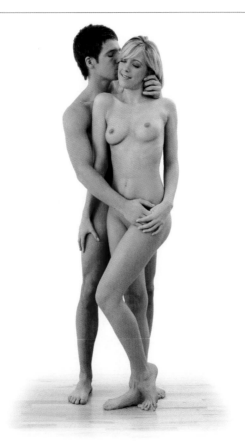

Tweak one ear lobe between your fingers, and nibble the other with your teeth.

Perfect for: Tantalizing one of her hottest erogenous zones.
Irresistible when: Accompanied by a whispered proposition.

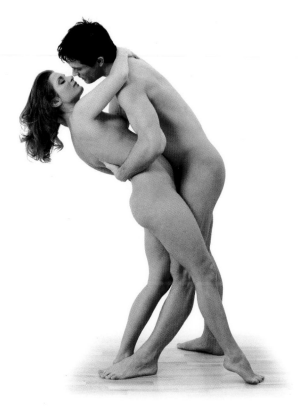

Take her in your arms like Rhett took Scarlett in *Gone with the Wind.*

Perfect for: Making her feel like a 1930s screen goddess.
Irresistible when: You pick her up, and whisk her off to bed.

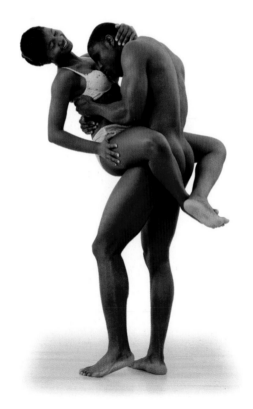

Lift her up, and sit her on your loins.

Perfect for: Making her feel the force of your desire.
Irresistible when: You press her against a wall, and ravish her with your mouth.

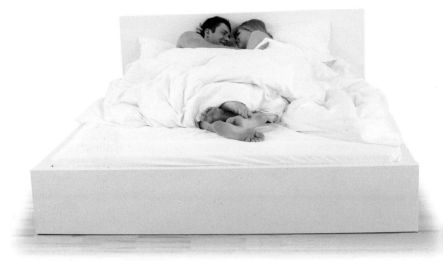

Get cuddly, and twine your feet around hers.

Perfect for: Smoochy intimacy when she can't get enough of you.
Irresistible when: You press foreheads, and nudge noses.

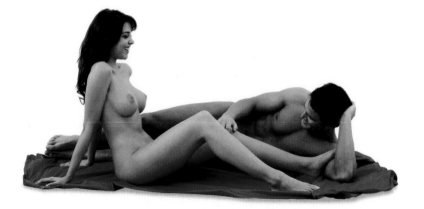

Lie at her feet, and tell her how gorgeous she's looking.

Perfect for: Making her feel like it's the first time, again.
Irresistible when: You explore her whole body with your eyes and fingertips.

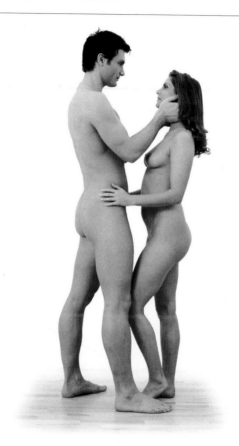

Cup her face tenderly in your hands.

Perfect for: "I love you" moments.
Irresistible when: You can't take your eyes off her.

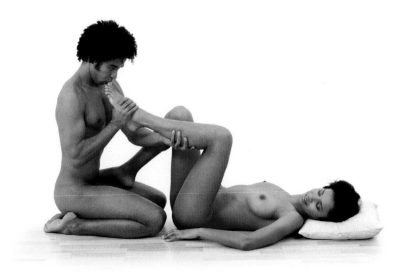

Slide her toes gently into your warm mouth.

Perfect for: The beginning of a mind-blowing foot massage.
Irresistible when: You let your teeth graze each toe.

Crooked caress

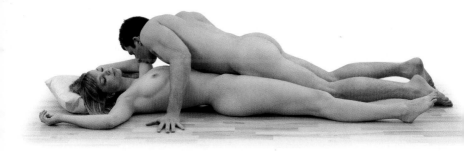

Flick the tip of your tongue across the sensual spot inside her elbow.

Perfect for: Tenderly disarming her.
Irresistible when: You nuzzle your way up, and kiss her sensitive underarm.

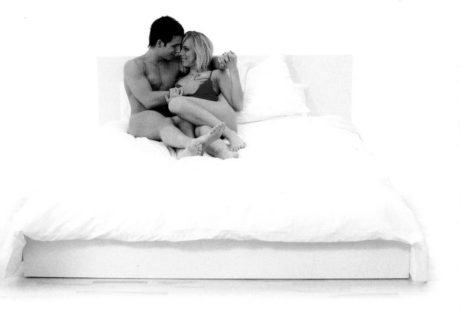

Let your hand wander into her bra during a sexy smooch.

Perfect for: The thrill of a teenage-style grope.
Irresistible when: You lavish her breasts with lip love too.

Novel seduction

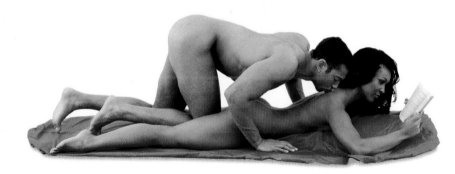

Interrupt her while she's reading by kissing her to distraction.

Perfect for: When playing hard to get makes her frisky.
Irresistible when: You invite her to touch your hardback.

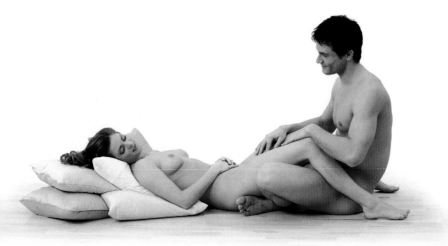

Stroke and caress the soft skin of her thighs.

Perfect for: Sending her into another dimension.
Irresistible when: You devote yourself to her sensual pleasure.

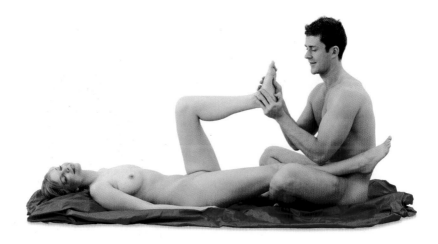

Move your fingers in deep circles on the sole of her foot.

Perfect for: When the way to her heart is through her feet.
Irresistible when: You finish by gently squeezing and twisting each toe in turn.

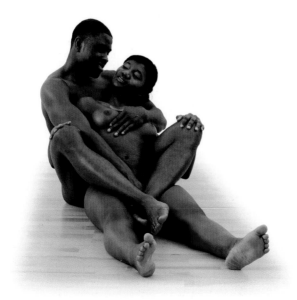

Twine your arms and legs around her in a koala-bear hug.

Perfect for: Sleepy, under-the-covers lust.
Irresistible when: She feels your boomerang is ready to nestle inside her.

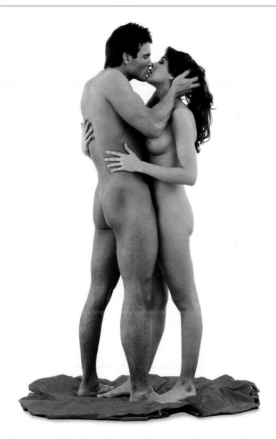

Grasp a soft fistful of her hair. Gently pull it as you kiss her.

Perfect for: Sending her into a sensual swoon.
Irresistible when: You savor the moment by hovering your lips on hers.

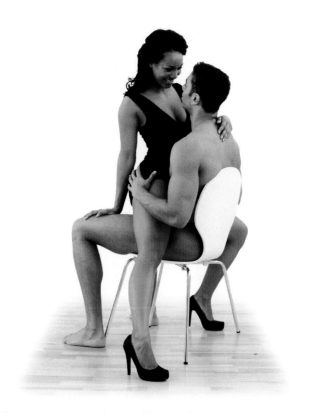

Smooth your hand along her thigh, pushing her dress up as you go.

Perfect for: Making her tingle as she feels your hot thighs on hers.
Irresistible when: You slide her dress over her hips, belly, waist, chest…

Pulling her softly

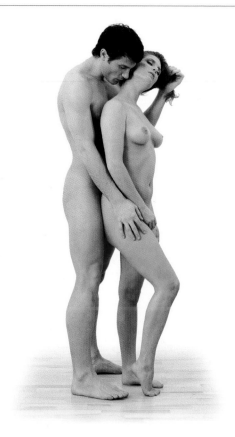

Twine her hair in your hand as you breathe softly on her neck.

Perfect for: Giving her goosebumps all over.
Irresistible when: You stroke her skin lightly with your fingertips.

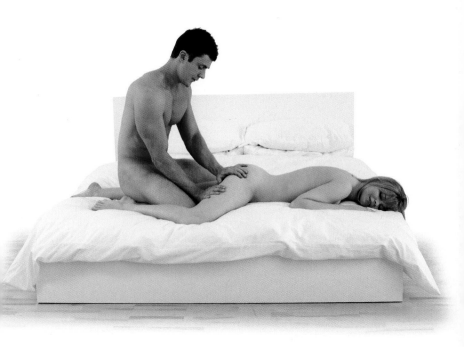

Give her a blissful massage by smoothing your thumbs along her thighs.

Perfect for: Taking away her tension.
Irresistible when: Your fingers stray fleetingly onto her pleasure palace.

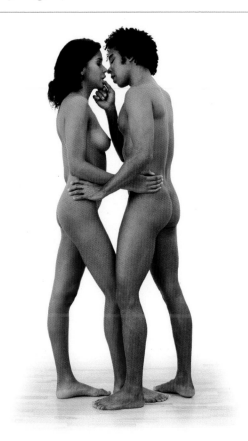

Squeeze her lower lip between thumb and forefinger before moving in to kiss her.

Perfect for: Creating delicious anticipation.
Irresistible when: You enclose her lower lip between yours, and suck gently.

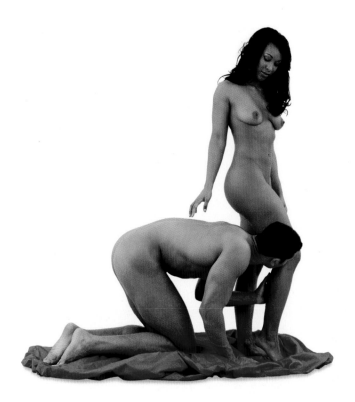

Give the backs of her knees a long, sexy kiss.

Perfect for: Giving her luscious leg trembles.

Irresistible when: You slide your palm ever so slowly along the inside of her thigh.

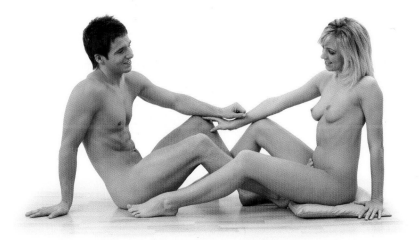

Find her clitoris with your toes, and wiggle them.

Perfect for: Under-the-table naughtiness in restaurants.
Irresistible when: You take her hand, and kiss it cheekily.

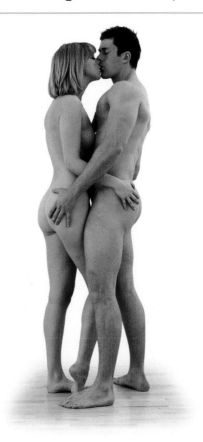

Move in for a kiss, and enclose her top lip in yours.

Perfect for: Amazing her with your kissing repertoire.
Irresistible when: You softly glide your tongue inside her lip.

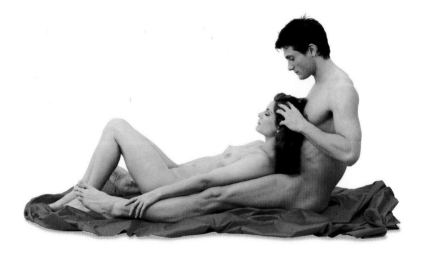

Move your fingers in slow, firm circles on her scalp.

Perfect for: Giving her a peak experience in the bathtub.
Irresistible when: You wrap her in a hot towel, and lead her to the bedroom.

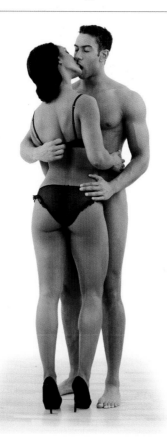

Kiss her passionately while sliding one hand around her back to unclasp her bra.

Perfect for: When she likes a stealthy but sure seduction.
Irresistible when: You fondle her breasts with cool, confident lust.

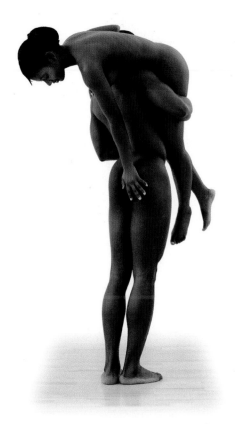

Take charge—pop her over your shoulder in a fireman's carry.

Perfect for: Giving her erotic, "I'm being taken" thrills.
Irresistible when: You lay her down on the bed in one fluid movement.

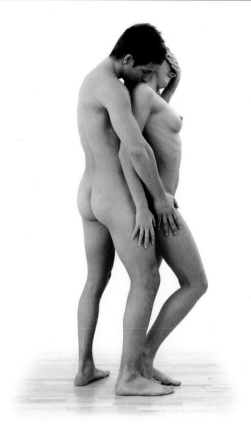

Surprise her by coming up from behind, covering her eyes, and nuzzling her neck.

Perfect for: A hot reunion when she's really missed you.
Irresistible when: Your hands go on tour.

Giving her some back-up

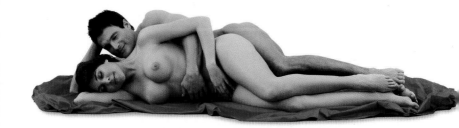

Hug her as you get cozy in spoons position.

Perfect for: Planting seeds of lust in her mind as she wakes up.
Irresistible when: You give her luxurious whole-body strokes.

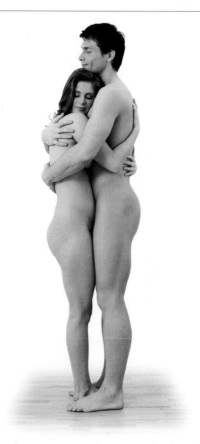

Enclose her in your arms, and press your body against hers.

Perfect for: Sweet reunions.
Irresistible when: You slide your hands down to her cheeks, and pull her in tight.

Naughty necking

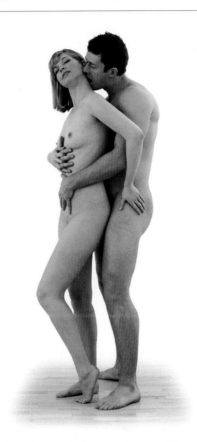

Seal your lips against her neck, and softly suck.

Perfect for: Thrilling her with the mark of your passion.
Irresistible when: You graze her shoulders and back with your hungry teeth.

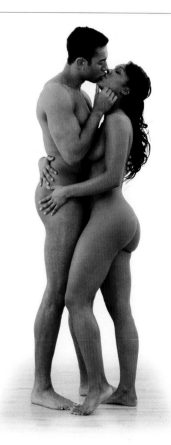

Turn her face up to yours, and put all your pent-up passion into a kiss.

Perfect for: Making her feel weak, wowed, and wooed.
Irresistible when: You breathlessly whisper your undying love.

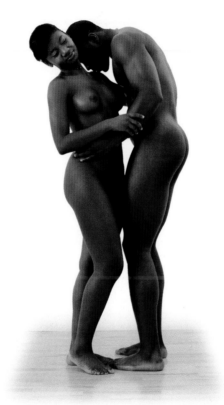

Trail sumptuous kisses along her collabone.

Perfect for: Setting this sensitive part of her body on fire.
Irresistible when: You stroke the small of her back with your hand as well.

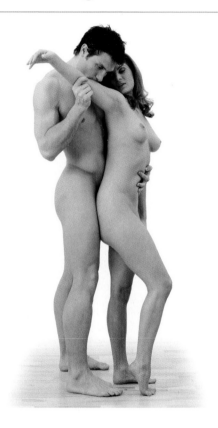

Plant a row of tender kisses along her arm.

Perfect for: An old-school seduction that will make her melt.
Irresistible when: You press your lips softly against the insides of her wrists.

Tiger touch

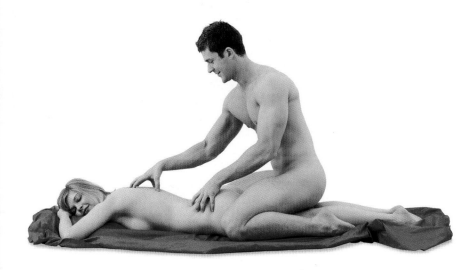

Massage her back with your hands in the shape of tiger claws.

Perfect for: When she's in the mood for something strong and predatory.
Irresistible when: You growl hungrily in her ear.

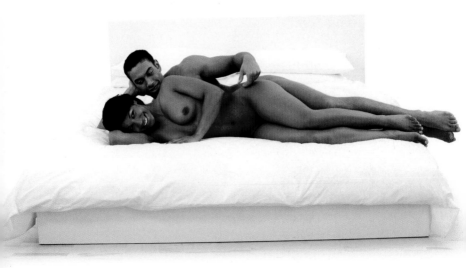

Cuddle up behind her, and draw the backs of your fingers over her skin.

Perfect for: A feathery touch that makes her shiver with lust.
Irresistible when: You leave no curve uncaressed.

Lust bite

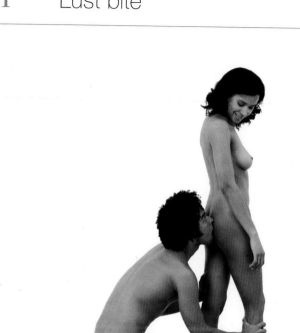

Give her cheek a sexy nibble.

Perfect for: Delighting her with your hungry passion.
Irresistible when: You lick her, and glide your teeth across her skin.

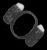

When the mood is rude and raunchy

Turn-ons to make her up for anything

When the mood is hot and erotic

Turn-ons to take her to passion paradise

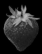

When the mood is sweet and sensual

Turn-ons to make her swoon

Q: What makes a woman truly enjoy sex?

A: Feeling thoroughly, tinglingly turned on beforehand. So turned on, in fact, that she can barely keep her trembling hands off your package. And so turned on that she can't stop a blissful "Mmmmmm" escaping from her lips.

And how do you achieve this?

Just turn the page. You'll find an eye-watering collection of turn-on techniques. Some are sweetly romantic. Others are sensual and erotic. Others are meant to make her giggle. And if she's filthy at heart, there's enough downright kinkiness and make-her-blush naughtiness to keep her happy for weeks.

Turn her on tonight like you've never turned her on before. Observe her mood and pick the turn-on that fits best. Or, as it's been said: tune in, turn on, and make out.

And… if you're fantasizing about being on the receiving end of a beautiful seduction, you can make it happen. Just close the book, flip it over, and hand it to your lover. She'll soon get the hint.

Contents

LONDON, NEW YORK, MELBOURNE, MUNICH, AND DELHI

Editor: Louise Frances
Designer: Alison Fenton
Project Editor: Laura Palosuo
Project Art Editor: Katherine Raj
Executive Managing Editor: Adèle Hayward
Managing Art Editor: Kat Mead
Production Editor: Kelly Salih
Production Controller: Alice Holloway
Creative Technical Support: Sonia Charbonnier
Art Director: Peter Luff
Publisher: Stephanie Jackson

First American Edition, 2009

Published in the United States by
DK Publishing
375 Hudson Street
New York, New York 10014

09 10 11 12   10 9 8 7 6 5 4 3 2 1

AD414—September 2009

Published in Great Britain by Dorling Kindersley Limited.

A catalog record for this book is available from the Library of Congress.

ISBN 978-0-7566-5444-3

DK books are available at special discounts when purchased in bulk for sales promotions,
premiums, fund-raising, or educational use. For details, contact: DK Publishing Special Markets,
375 Hudson Street, New York, New York 10014 or SpecialSales@dk.com.

Color reproduction by Colourscan, Singapore

Printed and bound in Singapore by Star Standard

Discover more at
www.dk.com

365

ways to turn her on

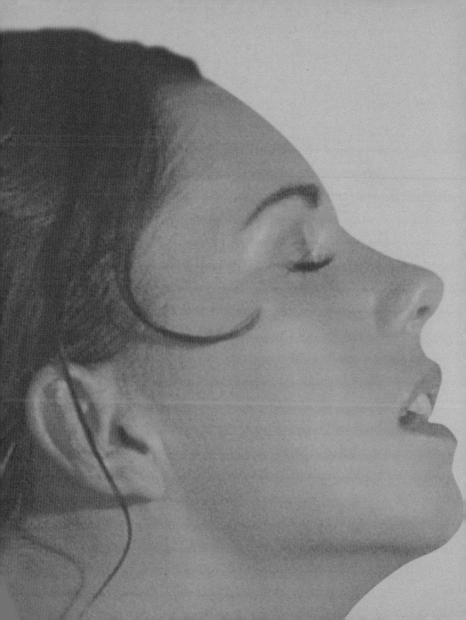

365

ways to turn her on